Recovery

For Elsevier:

Commissioning Editor: **Steven Black**

Development Editor: **Catherine Jackson**

Product Manager: **Gail Wright**

Designer: **Stewart Larking**

Illustration Manager: **Bruce Hogarth**

...fore the last date shown below.

F

A g

P

ME   te

Me
Me
Ser
Ips

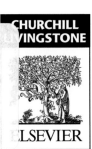

CHURCHILL
LIVINGSTONE
ELSEVIER

ISBN-13: 978-0-7506-8880-2

British Library Cataloguing in Publication Data
A catalogue record for this book is available from the British Library

Library of Congress Cataloging in Publication Data
A catalog record for this book is available from the Library of Congress

Note
Neither the Publisher nor the Author assume any responsibility for any loss or injury and/or damage to persons or property arising out of or related to any use of the material contained in this book. It is the responsibility of the treating practitioner, relying on independent expertise and knowledge of the patient, to determine the best treatment and method of application for the patient.

The Publisher

your source for books,
journals and multimedia
in the health sciences
www.elsevierhealth.com

Working together to grow
libraries in developing countries

www.elsevier.com | www.bookaid.org | www.sabre.org

ELSEVIER   BOOK AID
International   Sabre Foundation

The
Publisher's
policy is to use
**paper manufactured
from sustainable forests**

Printed in China

Contents

v

List of contributors

David Molan

I am on a journey of growth and healing that will continue for the rest of my days. Beyond the remit of the mental health system, I will work to share with others my knowledge of pathways to recovery. I enjoy and am grateful for every moment.

Janet Russell

I trained as an infant teacher and taught for several years. I've since had numerous jobs, ranging from civil servant to mental health support worker: all interspaced with periods of unemployment. My main interests are reading and creative writing. I am kept sane by creating and maintaining my garden, my great joy in life.

John McCloud

I qualified as an English teacher in 1988, worked briefly in secondary schools and then for an educational publisher for five years. For the last 10 years I have been a piano teacher. I am married with two children.

Emma

I'm Emma. I'm 32. I am a survivor.

Anna Last

I am a qualified librarian holding a BA(Hons) degree and an MA. I have previously worked at Suffolk College, Ipswich, and currently volunteer for the mental health charity MIND.

Dedication

For Gareth and Hywel

Introduction

*There are times in life when a person has to rush
off in search of hopefulness.*

Jean Giono

As we move further along the road into the 21st century, further into a post-modern era in which those guarantors of truth, science and religion, have lost some of their authority, a less credulous population no longer passively accepts an imperious psychiatric system that, at its worst, subjugates people into the role of patients and subdues their spirit along with their distress. What we need is a new way of looking at human distress that does not reduce suffering to neurotransmitter dysfunction; that does not dismiss the personal, phenomenological nature of distress by interpreting it according to the currently favoured model of psychological functioning; above all, one in which distress is not divorced from the social, cultural, political and ecological world occupied by the individual.

Forty years in the arena of mental health care has convinced me that there is no such thing as mental illness. There is no tangible, verifiable, classifiable 'it'. Yes, there is a form of human suffering that is experienced as a profound and disabling sadness and melancholy. Yes, there is a form of suffering in which people experience extraordinary states of consciousness and may lose their foothold in that broad band of a shared reality, with subsequent distress and disruption to their lives. But this is very different from an identifiable diagnosable 'it' called clinical depression or schizophrenia. I have come to believe that the language of psychiatry, in particular diagnostic terminology, must be discarded before any real progress is possible. Words such as 'psychosis' are the chains that shackle people to the psychiatric system. They are words that make compassionate care difficult. They are words that make it hard for people to recover a place for themselves in society. They are words that sustain stigma and discrimination. No wonder people resist being defined by these terms, loaded as they are with the projections of our darkest fears. To resist the label of schizophrenia, paranoid psychosis, schizoaffective disorder, is to my mind rational. Such resistance is more often seen as denial or lack of insight, but what is being denied is not the experiences themselves, which may be unusual, problematic and distressing, but the diagnostic conclusions.

The seminal work of the French philosopher Michel Foucault has provided a convincing analysis of the power of words. He argues that the language used by a powerful social group to objectify something soon becomes the dominant discourse and in time achieves the status of a truth even where this cannot be sustained by credible research. It can be seen as a way of appropriating power through 'expertise'. The language of psychiatric practice wraps human experience in a blanket of mystifying, excluding terminology, creating the role of expert – one who knows – and invalidating the personal subjective experience of the person seeking help who is consigned to the role of passive recipient of that 'expertise' (Foucault 1961).

What would happen if we were to discard Kraepelin's legacy and the ever widening net of psychiatric classification? What would happen if psychiatric terminology became as politically incorrect as sexist, racist and homophobic language? What would be the impact on people's identities and way of being in the world? What would be the risks? How would the practice of psychiatry change? One thing is certain – we would be forced to try and understand someone's troubled mind from the perspective of their lived experience and not from a medical or psychoanalytic framework. We would be forced to find an individual where he/she is and start the process of helping that individual to find ways of living in a less distressing, less problematic way from there. I do not pretend to have all the answers to these questions but my hope is that this book will contribute to the debate that is currently taking place in psychiatry around these themes.

During the latter half of the 20th century psychiatry transformed itself from a predominantly hospital-based service to a community-based service. But although you can take care out of the institution it is more difficult to take the institution out of care. Practices still exist which disempower people. Mental hospitals may have all but disappeared but the institution is still firmly ensconced within the mental health care system. Nevertheless, I fervently believe it is possible, as the first few decades of this century unfold, for psychiatry to transmute itself into a recovery-orientated mental health service.

It may seem from my introduction that this book is a throwback to the anti-psychiatry movement of the 1970s, when writers such as R.D. Laing and Thomas Szasz led a radical challenge to biomedical psychiatry. This is not the case. Rather, the book derives much of its inspiration from the challenge of the critical psychiatry movement, which, following its inception 25 years ago, has done much to deconstruct medical psychiatry and promote a robust and influential debate about alternatives (Bracken & Thomas 2001; Thomas & Bracken 2004). Essentially, critical psychiatry seeks to question the set of assumptions on which medical psychiatry is based and to highlight both its limitations and its potential to do harm. It seeks to loosen the conventions of practice and work collaboratively with service users to reconfigure services and widen ways of understanding and working with the 'experiential world of madness, alienation and distress'

(Thomas & Bracken 2004). Critical psychiatry stands at the forefront of campaigns to reduce the grip of pharmaceutical companies on psychiatry and to reduce the coercive elements in psychiatric practice.

The second major stimulus for the book comes from the consumer/survivor movement, which has created a powerful platform for the recovery experiences of people using mental health services which have challenged the therapeutic pessimism of previous decades. A number of anthologies of personal recovery stories have been published in recent years that signpost the way towards a growing sense of personal power, an unfolding of potential and sustained wellbeing, in spite of – and often because of – the vagaries of an untameable mind (Barker et al 1999; Read & Reynolds 2000; Barker & Buchanan Barker 2004; Gray 2006).

There are the beginnings of a paradigm shift in Britain away from a patient-centred, expert-led mental health service which has an orientation towards managing the symptoms of persistent and disabling disorders of the mind, towards a person-centred, collaboratively-led service that is orientated towards the recovery of wellbeing. Substantial long-term follow-up studies demonstrate that clinical and social recovery occurs in well over half of those people who have been hospitalised as the result of overwhelming psychological distress (Harding et al 1987; Harrison et al 2001). These studies lend support to an attitude of therapeutic optimism, providing evidence of a late recovery effect in many participants.

Criteria used to define 'recovery' in this research are exacting: they include evidence of work, an established social support network, no relapses for two years, and no longer taking antipsychotic medication. This is by no means the only definition of recovery, which for many has more to do with an acceptance and understanding of personal vulnerabilities and the development of strategies to minimise their impact. It is concerned with rebuilding identity, self-esteem and a fulfilling life. It is about recovering and sustaining wellbeing, sometimes in the context of continuing symptoms (Roberts & Wolfson 2004). In their guiding statement on recovery, the National Institute for Mental Health in England suggests a broad vision of recovery in which the focus is on 'the restoration, rebuilding, reclaiming or taking control of one's life' (NIMHE 2005). In the light of these wider definitions many people would argue that within a therapeutic culture of empowerment and hope, recovery is possible for the majority (Ahern & Fisher 2001).

In accord with my earlier stated position I have tried to write this book without recourse to diagnostic labels and the orthodox language of psychiatry, except where I am referencing other writers or referring directly to personal reflection on recovery material. Instead I have tried to capture something of the phenomenological nature of the experience of individuals in the outer reaches of distress. It is difficult for us as mental health professionals, steeped as we are in the medical tradition of psychiatry, to let go of these markers of practice. But I urge colleagues to try, to trust the capacity of people to find meaning in their distress and to make the life decisions that will ultimately lead to a less troubled way of being. People need substantial help in this process but it is my contention and experience that they will be helped more effectively by a committed person-centred practitioner who is prepared to make that journey of discovery and recovery with them than the patient-centred practitioner who offers prescriptive solutions. One of the releasing aspects of this approach is in not knowing – not knowing what has gone wrong for this person in their life; not knowing what to do about it. But what a privilege and how worthwhile it is to collaborate with that person in finding out.

The second point I want to make about language is to say that I have used the inclusive 'us' and 'we' extensively in the text. It may at times seem uncertain to whom I am addressing my arguments – people using mental health services, mental health professionals or Everyman. My focus has intentionally been inclusive, as I believe the recovery process is a universal one and the themes explored in this book are relevant to us all. We mental health professionals can no longer think of ourselves as a 'subspecies' endowed with immunity from the dilemmas, adversities and suffering of the rest of humanity. We cannot act in a way that seems to deny our human vulnerability and our need to recover and sustain our own wellbeing. Daniel Fisher, a psychiatrist whose own experience of 'madness' has led him to becoming a passionate and influential voice in the recovery through empowerment movement in America, identifies in his recovery story a need for his therapist to 'be a real person' for him (Fisher 1999). We have to be real in our contact with people. We have our wounds. We seek our own roads to recovery and the more aware and openly we travel the more help we are likely to be to fellow travellers.

The book is not derived solely from my professional experience of psychiatry over the past 40 years but also from my own struggle for psychological survival and recovery. There has been something of a trend for authors in the mental health field to 'come out' in recent years and I have found this book impossible to write without a profound examination of my own journey. I hope the inclusion of aspects of my personal story will not be seen as an indulgence but will, along with the other personal testimonies, add some authenticity and validity to what I have to say in the wider text.

Chapter 1, 'In search of sanity', addresses the question of how to be sane in an increasingly insane world. As the incidence of psychiatric morbidity in Britain continues to rise along with prescriptions for psychotropic drugs, there is an urgent need for us to reflect on our egoistic, consumer-orientated lifestyles and discover a way of being that is more compatible with health.

Chapter 2 considers 'The nature of human distress'. While the medicalisation of distress can bring relief, it is always at some cost. The deleterious effects of even the newer, 'cleaner' antipsychotic drugs are well known and the stigma associated with psychiatric labelling widely testified to. But more than this, pathologising distress creates the illusion of a morbid psychobiological dysfunction that can only be resolved by expert intervention, thus sowing the seed of passive vulnerability. By way of contrast, the chapter sets out to make the case for seeing states of psychological overwhelm as having meaning in the context of a person's lived experience. It is through decoding that meaning that people are empowered to regain a state of wellbeing.

Chapter 3, 'Roads to recovery', is the core of the book. I have drawn on the mythology of the hero's journey as the format for discussing the recovery from overwhelming, troubled states of mind. This is not done in a whimsical way but in the sincere belief that the journey through 'madness', which is often long and arduous, brings forth the heroic qualities of an individual.

Chapter 4 discusses 'The family dimension of recovery'. Ignoring John Donne's dictum that 'no man is an island', psychiatry has almost exclusively focused on the individual. It postulates some dysfunction within, to be treated or resolved, largely ignoring the family system and the wider community as both a cause of distress and a source of healing.

Chapter 5 considers the important 'Cultural and community dimension of recovery'. Many mental health service consumers and survivors have testified to the fact that overcoming the stigma and marginalisation that accompany psychiatric diagnoses is more difficult than recovering from the initial dysfunction. Yet the collective voice of the psychiatric professions is strangely muted in the political arena of life. The chapter is a clarion call to colleagues to be more voluble in confronting the many social injustices and inequalities that are so often at the root of disabling distress and make recovery an obstacle course.

Chapter 6 explores 'The spiritual dimension of recovery'. In this secular age we have relegated the spiritual, transcendent way of being to a place of minor significance in our lives. But increasingly we are recognising that the values we live by and the hedonistic and materialistic lifestyles we pursue do not sustain authentic happiness. There is, endemic in Western society, a malaise and ennui, born out of spiritual hunger, which often underlies human distress. The quest for wellbeing must be holistic in its scope and encompass the spiritual dimension.

Chapter 7 looks at 'The creative dimension of recovery'. At the heart of humankind is a propensity for creativity – how else would we have survived and prospered so successfully as a species? This creative energy strengthens the spirit and gives vitality, vibrancy and meaning to life. For many people artistic endeavour is a key element in the recovery of wellbeing.

Chapter 8, the final chapter of the book, focuses on 'Recovery relationships'. As part of the family of *Homo sapiens* we are interdependent by nature and that interdependence is never more apparent than when mental adversity descends disruptively on our lives. It is the empathetic care we receive from others that offers safe mooring as we struggle to avoid being overwhelmed by troubled waters. Of all the facets of the recovery process it is the catalytic effect of caring relationships that enables us to move forward in our quest for wellbeing.

Interspersed between the chapters of the book are five recovery stories generously and courageously contributed by people I have come to know professionally

5

and personally. They represent the soul of the book, reflecting the indomitable spirit in human nature that sustains people in their struggle for survival and recovery in the face of turmoil and disintegration. They map the road less travelled – that uniquely individual road to recovery, taken after a period of being lost and despairing in a bewildering inner world. David Molan talks about his quest for wellbeing through a process of intuitive self-healing. This has involved detoxifying the physical, emotional and spiritual domains of his life and the extensive use of holistic therapies. Janet Russell describes her journey of recovery, after being hospitalised for several years, as a process of self-empowerment and self-realisation which has enabled her to transcend continuing symptoms of distress. John McCloud explains how he confronted the need to give up his addictive highs and avoid his incapacitating lows, after several rollercoaster years of wildly fluctuating moods, finding a life worth living in the process. Emma describes how, after years of emotional turmoil and self-harm, she eventually found the strength to deal with early trauma and the 'everyday lacerations of the spirit' to find meaning and purpose in her life. Anna Last relates how she became lost in a labyrinthine depression which undermined her confidence and dismantled her life. She describes how the green shoots of her recovery grew out of creative writing.

The book is a distillation of experience and reflection gathered during my working life, which began in the institutional world of mental hospitals and has continued in the dynamism of community mental health services. It is an enormous privilege to have been a companion to so many people on their recovery journeys; to have been with them in the landscape of their lives, through difficult terrain and onto the uplands where sure-footed progress can be made. As the discerning reader will become aware, the book is written 'on the shoulders of giants'. The work of humanistic therapists, philosophers and educators Carl Rogers and John Heron has had a profound effect on my personal and working life. The ideas of radical psychiatrists R.D. Laing and Peter Breggin and the vision of my nursing colleague Professor Phil Barker have provided deep sources of inspiration. The published writing of survivors and consumers of the psychiatric system, particularly Ron Coleman and Patricia Deegan, have continually challenged me to think beyond convention. I also owe a debt of gratitude to my colleagues in the Ipswich Outreach Team who over the past seven years have exemplified the practice out of which the contents of this book have arisen.

Finally my heartfelt thanks to my partner, Ann, who has patiently and generously given her time to help me refine the text and again to Ann, to Bron, Gemma and Jan who have been such a healing presence in my life during a time when I have been careworn and laden with grief.

In search of sanity

1

Our real journey in life is interior; it is a matter of growth, of deepening, of an ever greater surrender to the creative action of love and grace in our hearts. Never was it more necessary to respond to that action.

Thomas Merton

Introduction

The current political and personal agenda in Western culture is dominated by egotism and consumerism. We have never been 'better off', and yet the incidence of psychological distress is at an all time high. At any one time, one sixth of adults in Britain are experiencing dysfunctional levels of distress (Office of National Statistics 2000a). The premise of this chapter is that we have lost touch with our true being, become dislocated from our place in the world, and in doing so have sought meaning in acquisition. What we have in terms of money, status, material possessions has become the way in which we define ourselves and measure the quality and worth of our lives. Small wonder, then, that there is continuing anxiety associated with preserving what we have and a desperate need to acquire more. The theme of this chapter is not one that advocates the philosophy of austerity, but one that counsels against investing what we have with so much meaning, what the psychoanalyst and philosopher Erich Fromm has called the 'having mode of existence'.

· · · · · · · · · · ·

Many people are now recognising that the pathway to a more sustainable sense of wellbeing is to be found in a more aware, reflective, altruistic, spiritually conscious way of life. Beyond the ego, in the heart and soul of humankind, is a capacity for loving kindness, for experiencing the joy of existence and a profound sense of our connectedness with others and every living thing. Sadly it is often through 'suffering that we are able to make this transition towards a '*being mode*' of existence' (Fromm 1976). To live in the '*being mode*' means to give expression to our most noble attributes, our talents and faculties. It means to renew oneself, to grow, to love, to imagine, to contemplate, to be present in the here and now. To live in the '*being mode*' requires us to let go of the objects of desire as our primary source of meaning and fulfilment and instead to re-focus our attention on the unfolding of our potential as persons, on our need for relatedness and oneness with the world around. It is that process of becoming the person we truly are that is the source of aliveness, security and wellbeing. Psychological and somatic symptoms can be seen as metaphors which carry the message that our way of being in the world is incompatible with wellness. If we can see the meaning in these messages and learn from the innate wisdom of the body/mind, we can move from breakdown to breakthrough in our mental health.

We live in a strange world in which we are bombarded by imagery that extols the '*having mode*' of existence, doing work that diminishes and exhausts us; a world in which our rapacious, hedonistic pursuit of travel, acquisition and entertainment offers us only transient satisfaction. We load our personal relationships with the expectation that these unions will make us whole and our lives complete, only to abandon them when that illusion is inevitably shattered. We educate our children in a way that gives them a knowledge base that is wide and often deep, but teaches them little about how to live. Our attitude towards the earth remains arrogant and exploitative while the threat of an environmental apocalypse becomes the spectre of our future. I would argue that it is our society that is bewildered and bewildering and the sanest among us are those who recognise that their distress is a symptom of a dysfunctional sociopolitical system, a system that continues to promote a way of life incompatible with wellbeing.

8

It seems entirely plausible that the medicalisation of depression, a condition endemic in contemporary Western society, serves to deflect attention away from these political and social conditions which undermine mental health. To follow where the symptoms of depression lead would take us to all that is dispiriting in modern life, but instead we attempt to cure it with antidepressant drugs on the grounds that profound states of unhappiness are biologically based. Hillman (1976), in his treatise on re-visioning psychology, argues that everyone, at times, experiences psychopathology, for that is the language of the psyche in extremis, and that rather than seeking to alleviate our symptoms we should contemplate their meaning as a basis for social action and cultural change.

'Attention! Attention!' These are the first words the protagonist in Aldous Huxley's last novel, the Utopian fantasy 'Island', hears as he regains consciousness, having survived a shipwreck. He finds himself cast away on an island that has remained isolated from the infective culture of the rest of the world. The book describes a society that perpetuates a more virtuous and ethical way of life. The fundamental message of the book – the urgent need to wake up, to have more of our attention free for living – is more pertinent now than when it was first published, more than forty years ago.

The first crucial step in changing our way of being in the world is to increase awareness. To be more alive, moment to moment, to the flow of experience, to what we are sensing, thinking, feeling, intuiting, doing. It is this deepening awareness that reconnects us with the essence of our being, with others and with the natural and cosmic world. It re-acquaints us with the purpose of living – what Hillman has referred to as 'the development of a more soulful life'. This may sound somewhat esoteric, but it is neither less nor more than our natural heritage, a manifestation of our being that only seems alien because we have become so distant from it. The influential psychologist and philosopher Carl Rogers, in his reflections on the nature of man, describes how an enriched and meaningful life can be derived from an 'increasing openness to experience' (Rogers 1961). If we can live with less defensiveness so that experience, whether from within or from the world around us, is fully lived rather than denied or distorted, then we will begin to feel more alive, more in touch with our essential self. This can take courage because it can confront us with painful feelings, base motives and destructive inclinations. But it is only through this soul searching that our capacity for loving kindness, affiliation and ethical living unfolds. It is this mindful living that increasing numbers of people now seek through counselling, spiritual practice and eco-consciousness.

Thomas Berry, in his writing on eco-consciousness, reflects on how dislocated we humans have become from our place in the natural world (Berry 1999); how our arrogance has led us to the delusion that we have a God-given right to dominion over all things. We continue to exploit and pollute the earth at will in order to sustain an affluent Western lifestyle, to the point where reparative action would only be possible if there were to be a fundamental change in our cultural preoccupations. So far, our political, corporate, educational and religious institutions have failed to provide the vision or to generate the dynamism to help heal the world. A new way of interacting with the earth must evolve if humankind is to survive; this new way can emerge if we rediscover the wonder, the celebration and respect for the community of life of which we are a part. Berry talks about 'the great work', 'the heroic quest' that faces us over the coming decades if we are to step back from ecological catastrophe. The impetus for this 'great work' will not come solely from visionary leadership, but as a result of the reverberations from our damaged world that are already manifesting themselves in the increasing incidence of psychological and physical malaise. More and more people in search of wellbeing are beginning to recognise the need to harmonise human existence with the natural world. We must return to a reverence for nature, not in any romantic sense but in a way that acknowledges that we are part of nature, part of the ecosystem of this planet on which we depend. John Clare, the 19th century nature poet, became irrevocably lost in a melancholic delusional world as the countryside with which he felt such a close affinity was enclosed and his freedom to commune with it restricted. How much more so are we affected, disconnected as we are from the earth that sustains us.

If we are living with awareness the preoccupations of the ego become less of a concern and the ego becomes what it is, a mutable persona in which guise we strut the stage of everyday life. Think for a moment what it might mean to be less ego-driven. We would not be so anxiously concerned about the presentation of self in everyday life, about embellishing the ego with possessions and status, about conforming slavishly to the prevailing social mores. Our self-esteem would not be so dependent on the approbation of others or on acquiring the outward symbols of success but would derive from a deeper source. We would not be so driven to achieve for achievement's sake but would be energised by selfless motives. If we were less egocentric, we would not be so entranced with ourselves and instead would be rightfully entranced by the world of which we are but a part. In this egoless way of being, jealousy, resentment, fear, depression, blame, failure, hopelessness and guilt would not well up in our consciousness and disturb our equilibrium so frequently.

I do not mean to suggest that the quest for happiness lies in the dissolution of the ego – in Western culture we prize individualism too much for that to happen. What I am proposing is a less egocentric form of individualism, a way of being that is not ego-led but is an expression of the authentic self in which the heart and soul of humankind is set free. Living with more openness leads, in Rogers' view, to what he calls *existential living* – we are more in the moment as that experience flows through us, more freely responsive to whatever we discover there. It is this deeper self that leads us towards a more joyful, compassionate, ethical way of being. This contrasts with the behavioural rigidity with which we habitually interact with the world.

It might seem that the 'freedom to be' is a licence for selfishness and the unfettered expression of the shadow side of our nature. In fact the reverse is true – the more our life is centred around the '*having mode*' of existence, the more it is ego led, and the more self-gratifying and lacking in regard for others our behaviour is likely to become. Rogers placed great store by what he saw as the affiliative nature of humankind – our need to connect, relate and belong. His conviction, drawn from a lifetime study of people and their quest for wellbeing, was that in the process of unfolding our potential we naturally move in the direction of constructive social engagement (Rogers 1961). The more we know of ourselves the better able we are to trust the rightness of our actions and interactions. Like many people I find it difficult to square this with the malevolence, atrocity and antisocial acts we witness every day on our television screens and on our streets. But as the philosopher and theologian Paul Tillich suggests, such acts represent an estrangement from our essential nature – a separation from our self, from our neighbour and from God (Tillich 2000). Tillich takes an optimistic view of human nature, believing that we can recover the path and return to a state of grace:

> Grace strikes us when we are in great pain and restlessness. It strikes us when we walk through the dark valley of a meaningless empty life. It strikes us when we feel our separation is deeper than usual because we have violated another life, a life which we loved or from which we were estranged. (p. xii)

Central to the nature of being human is the quest to make sense of our experience and make meaningful life choices in response to that experience of reality.

Processing experience is something that largely occurs in the relational context. We make sense of experience not only through an internal mental process, but also through interaction with others and through our cultural heritage. Any disruption of this capacity to process experience appropriately inevitably leads to distress and dysfunction. It is not difficult to surmise how, as the result of unfavourable attachment experience and trauma in early life, distortions arise in our ways of viewing ourselves and the world. It is these difficulties in processing experience accurately, carried forward into adult life, that lead to troubled and overwhelmed states of mind. If we do not learn emotional competence, then we are vulnerable to being emotionally overwhelmed, and if our emergent self is not accepted and prized then it is likely that we will be confused about how to be in the world and will find it difficult to value ourselves. Wellbeing is dependent on the fundamental belief that *I'm okay and you're okay* – a psychological formulation of the Christian ethic *love your neighbour as yourself.*

There is no such thing as perfection in the affairs of humankind: perfection belongs only to the gods. In our struggles to actualise more of our qualities and potentials we will fall short. Few reach the goal of becoming what Rogers referred to as 'fully functioning human beings'. But we can nevertheless aspire to achieving that goal, and we can engage in that process of realising our potential and thus make *being* rather than *having* the central goal of our lives.

Insane labels – a personal reflection on recovery

David Molan

It is strange to assign beginnings to something as elusive as one's state of mind, so a hospital admission seems an arbitrary enough starting point. Indeed, by definition, it is when my problems began. Six years ago, while studying at university, I embarked on my journey through the mental health system. I had thought my path though life would take a rather different course to the one I have followed since. Initially I was given a diagnosis of drug induced psychosis. This was followed by such insane labels as manic depression, schizoaffective disorder, schizophrenia – in fact combinations of labels, as many and as varied as the ever growing DSM criteria and the creative minds of psychiatrists would allow.

The systems of psychiatry as I have encountered them and my chosen route have diverged widely. The belief in my inherent genetic dysfunction and supposed chemical imbalance (neither of which have any conclusive supporting evidence) leading to my present diagnoses confers a sentence beyond all rationale. With 'incurable prospects', I may only expect 'remission'. My own health philosophy is grounded in a more holistic approach; this is the only one that has made any sense to me in my search for health. Experimentation and an open outlook, both an absolute necessity, have borne successful health outcomes in a climate that would have me sceptical. Special individuals, who penetrate the surface of my world, forming the substance of my health findings, have influenced my daily practices, outlooks and lifestyle.

Various people have reacted to me in a plethora of remarkable ways. Surprisingly, I have found that those with no experience of 'mental health' except their own worldliness have had a dramatic impact on me, often bringing gems of insight and groundedness. Within the context of the health system, I have, with reflection, gained a view of the good hearts and intentions of all those concerned. It is the phenomenal heritage of confusion about mental health, the misplaced beliefs from our recent social and medical past, acted out daily in encounters with patients and public, that now concerns me. My desire is that those left acting out misplaced prejudices within the hospitals and the wider system be educated or move on.

I find myself less confused these days, though paradoxically less certain about life than before my adventure began. I have found a matured home in my heart and a confidence in my step, gaining openness to the mystery of life and the limitations of my logical mind. Health is a state of one's present relationship to self and environment. Mine is currently rather good. I find myself settled, my days full of moments that bring me happiness and on a path set on overcoming any possible criteria of ill health.

When the hospital system took apparent charge of my mind, the signs that my relationship to my environment was poor had been brewing for a while. Parts of my inner world were bizarrely reflected in my social mirror; my wit to deal with this in a fitting manner was simply inadequate. I perceived the nature of the situation to some degree. I attempted to communicate it in a variety of ways and found only exasperation in my friends and in professionals. What was happening was outside of my previous experience; I wanted to express it, to play with it, live it, and to have a space to hold on to it. I suddenly found myself inappropriate in my environment, where others were preparing for exams. I did not know where to go, or how to travel, so instead found myself taken to hospital.

My reaction, lacking in overt volition, did serve the purpose of moving me to a position within life that is far closer to my soul's desires. I succumbed to following the expression of inner voices or high-spirited emotional horses, leading me to a plateau of peace and a vision of beauty. This seems to conflict with the initial, subsequent and somewhat continuing reaction of the 'medical model forces' to suppress, dampen and expel these yearnings. Potent drugs from the burgeoning pharmacopoeia were ultimately given as the panacea for all my perceived ills. Improvements in my outlook were ascribed to the medications working; any detrimental change as a need to review my medication. Any request to stop the prescribed drugs was met with a response that strongly underlined the incredible risk involved, backed by copious graphs and pharmaceutical sponsored studies, illustrating the dire prognosis for such a course of action. The desire to move away from the harsh poisons was taken as indicative of my illness and of my lack of insight into my own condition, undermining any of my points of view expressed in my own words rather than jargon. It is understandable to have such strong and unwavering belief in chemical means to therapeutic ends, given that the theory that states of mind are mediated by purely physical and organic routes gave birth to the discipline of psychiatry.

Doom-laden predictions of my future, based on questionable studies claiming complete recovery is an elusive goal for the majority, have melted in their importance. I choose the positive anecdotes of the minority who have come through and have shown the way as my destiny. I continue to believe that recovery is possible for all. My path has taken me away from the medical model. Health is the presence of vibrant wellbeing rather than the absence of symptoms. My daily experience of intuitive self-healing has provided too great an evidence base to be dismissed, to the point where wellbeing is a natural result of my own adapting and developing awareness. Surely true health is in our very nature!

It takes an inordinate effort to prevent ourselves returning to alignment with health. Toxic diets lead to absurd degrees of imbalance. Mass consumption of alcohol, sugar, caffeine, allopathic and recreational drugs undermines holistic health. The harbouring of toxic emotions and the suppression of our natural spirit can cause our inner creativity to stagnate for want of expression. The incredible concept of loneliness on an over-populated planet leads to confusion, doubt of our own worth and place, starving our intrinsic need of community and communing.

Have we reached the point where talking to ourselves, our higher selves, has become a reason for scorn? It is our inner dialogue that charts our course through life within this world. Could it be that when this is awry in individuals, the collective suffers? Healing is called for on a global scale and when we heal our individual pains, global healing is inevitable. We affect our environment! Moving away from suppression and on to a view of our innate beauty and wellness is so important. My experiential view is that pathways to recovery are innately present; in fact, given the inclination, we can maximise these natural processes and create them ourselves. As we take each step, we craft our own.

My travels have brought me through territories that only seem familiar now. They have been made my own through exploration. Engaging with the journey has taken some courage; fear has certainly been present as I was given an overriding lack of choice of ways towards recovery. It is this that has led me on to solutions, discoveries and insights, reinforcing my view of an innate healing inclination. I am now grasping why these alternatives to the tablets had to be won by trial and error. It would have been so much gentler to have had realisations presented at the beginning, when I was vulnerable and in need of solutions and help rather than the shock of lock, key, injections, and grandiose clinical references to my faulty genetics. The fact is allopathic psychiatrists did not know what they were doing, nor understand the essence of my, or many of my fellow travellers', experiences. They looked at me as an objective condition, cared, but at the same time remaining distanced. This is ridiculous, this is a human condition – to 'cut out' some mysterious invasive disorder would have been to cauterise and remove part of my soul crying out in pain. There would be silence in the doped aftermath, no response to the question in my symptoms, no transition towards real health, just suppression and control.

Depression and mania are natural responses to the highs and lows of life internalised, seeking expression. Schizophrenia is a natural response to our inner voices and guides' messages, warped by continual refusal to acknowledge them. Symptoms may be dealt with in a socially acceptable manner without our sacred space being violated, learning, in the process, to live with each other and ourselves in harmony.

My own tools have involved an expansive collection of methods that are repeatable by anyone with the inclination. I took a view of myself as having a high concentration of emotional energy in my system and by discharging it through tears, song or primal noise would release states of grief and anger in a structured and functional manner. I did this by taking myself into a special place to allow their expression, where they would not be misinterpreted as being current in their association, but accepted for what they are: natural feelings that have been deferred or delayed. In this context they can be allowed to run their course in a most pleasant way, leaving me feeling purified. This seems to be removing the causative factors, leaving me with long-term emotional stability. Now I find fewer emotional states or moods crystallising from the seeds of circumstances. Both my mind and my physical health have recovered, showing me that the storing of emotions can lead to an inner concentration of toxins on a cellular level. Renewed clarity of inner vision reveals the effectiveness of this process to me. The real and lasting experience of freshness of spirit coincides with my reclaiming parts of my memory, character and youthful aspirations, I can only relate to soul retrieval, or catharsis.

My physical detoxification takes several forms. A two-day liver cleanse removes the stored chemicals that my system has ingested, particularly in the form of past medications, recreational drugs and modern diet, which has a profound effect on my overall vitality. This has had a large impact on my present moment awareness and ability to move on from my past, letting go of my waste matter on a physical, emotional and mental level. Joining classes has given me regular access to yoga, salsa dancing, chi gung, massage, shiatsu and reflexology. These have impacted on my self-awareness through the mind–body connection. The benefits of healing with others as fellow individuals are immeasurable. The lack of focus on classic clinical criteria has allowed my perception to realign to a far calmer balance and outlook.

My diet has a dramatic impact on my mood and state of mind. As my health has improved, so has my sensitivity to the consequences of this incredibly potent form of medicine, moving me past the need for nicotine, caffeine and more. Similarly, my consumption of information has changed. Random television, with its fast food feast of low quality, highly stimulating ultraviolet bathing, has been replaced by a more refined and rarefied selection of edifying film and theatre. The habitual consumption of poisonous and strongly emotive daily newspapers and other publications have been replaced by word of mouth as a gentler informer of current affairs, offering positive choice of focus to raise my ambient emotional climate. Spoken word recordings ranging through self-development, astronomy and languages have given me ready access to a stable voice and structure and the constant availability of mentors. I have used these by contemplating the words of the orator, repeating the words out loud and modelling them, or just as background sound to subtly influence my state. This gives value to every moment of the day where my inner thoughts might otherwise be given to idling or free rein through rough territory. The balance of dialogue in my day has been heavily weighted now towards intelligent, uplifting content.

A digital dictaphone has enabled me to record my own voice and conversation with others, naturally with their permission. Playing these later has often reflected a dramatically different interpretation of the dialogue. This has developed the ability in me to have another point of view in every interaction. Positive reading material concerned with health and growth is my current priority. Putting this into practice has involved real time confrontation with habits and the innate process of changing them. Times of transition were made far easier through understanding their nature, particularly in relation to withdrawal symptoms from medications. By reading material that explained this, symptoms could be dealt with practically rather than worried about.

Social choices have become more discerning, leading to relationships that are nutritious for all concerned and with a consciousness of how each person is appropriate in different ways. Adopting certain personal rules of conversation and interaction has given me far more freedom and security in meeting and working with others while adjusting to my renewed self.

My choice of inner play has changed and is now filled with questions and processes that lead me to a daily feeling of excitement and enjoyment rather than ruminations over past discussions or perceived failures. This springs from a knowledge that there is a limit of focus at any given moment, so, with that choice available, why choose anything other than beliefs that serve you now and outlooks that promote wellbeing?

Through all this a connection with some seat of 'beautiful sanity' within me has become apparent in a form of writing that developed. I learnt to touch type at the computer. I found that I would start writing with no active construction. Realisation of my words and sentence structure came later. In the time it took to type them, pages of text would appear as if by dictation, that in retrospect made an inordinate amount of sense. This has become a readily accessible means of contacting my source or the part of myself that knows the right answers for me. I recognised that all of us have a reservoir in our subconscious that houses every experience, word, feeling, and it can be accessed given the right stimulus. By stepping out of the way and allowing a means for this immense natural intelligence to speak, my writing and inner voice have overridden a fear of my rebellious psyche that was fed to me. All the words and language that have emerged have been supporting and loving.

These findings and practices now seem like common sense and are part of my every day. I do remember a time when most things seemed bizarre, outlandish and certainly not to be acted upon or discussed, but, given how health enhancing they have proved to be, no wonder I went awry. Realising the value of these lessons has been my best investment.

Initial hospital admissions were preceded by hallucinations, wondrous auras of light surrounding people and subtle meanings to music and nature. When perceived to be awry, visions are classified in a clinical manner, rather than acknowledged as a source of true wealth drawn from a broader vision of reality. In their context mine were disturbing to the psychiatrist who saw me and led to a medical and isolative treatment. Since recovering my balance and entering a course of studies aligned with healing, my peer group welcomes my viewpoint and my experiences alluded to above have become stronger, more grounded. This has reinforced my outlook that these experiences are an aspect of healthy function, to be nurtured, sharing the ways in which we use these as tools. The old healing arts may be outside of a cumbersome ill handled scientific view of reality, yet those who subscribe to them confirm their usefulness repeatedly. Who needs the statistical reports? When you've experienced massage, you know it works.

Our innate intelligence is here to be tapped and utilised as a resource. Ignorance of that becomes problematic for some. Our outer and inner worlds are reflections: they have to be – how could it be another way? Observe our circles of madness. The way we maltreat our water supplies, of which we are 80% composed, yet expect immunity from the effects. Under the guise of technological advancement we pump toxins into the air that we breathe. Look at the way our Earth, shared by a small family of 6 billion or so, is being dishevelled like an unruly teenager's bedroom. Repercussions are inevitable unless we mature as individuals and a global community. Ill omens of disease are signs to our little minds of the vast importance of awakening to our big mind. Supporting those who are emotionally sensitive, can we move towards sharing a happy dream for generations to come? The walls we build are so thin, giving the illusion of separation. There are networks of able-minded individuals connecting globally today; we are one step closer to linking constructively. Whatever the role played within this unfolding play of health system creation, your part is valuable.

I have remained without chemical or hospital intervention of any sort since leaving hospital. Today I am working towards healing goals in the mental health arena, helping others to walk their own pathways to recovery.

The nature of
human distress

2

We are our own question mark.

R.D. Laing

Introduction

This chapter explores alternative ways of understanding the experience of the human distress and suffering that bring people into contact with mental health services. Central to this exploration is the conviction that while the experience of mental dis-ease may be profoundly disabling and problematic for the individual and society, it does not represent a pathological discontinuity separating it from ordinary human experience. I want to make the case for de-medicalising severe distress primarily because I have come to believe that for the majority of people, having one's mental anguish attributed to a pathological process is profoundly unhelpful. Diagnostic terms such as psychosis shackle people to the psychiatric system. They are terms that sustain stigma and discrimination and make it hard for people to recover a place for themselves in the mainstream of life. To be 'diagnosed' can be an assault on one's identity and a disempowering experience that takes away much of the personal responsibility for recovery and invalidates any attempt to understand distress in the context of the individual's lived experience. No wonder so many people resist diagnostic labels that threaten to eclipse their whole identity and place a straitjacket on their lives.

A review of studies of public opinion around the world reveals that despite the grip of medical psychiatry and the pharmaceutical industry on mental health services, most people reject biological theories of mental dysfunction, placing much more emphasis on psychosocial factors (Read & Haslam 2004). I recognise that many people find relief in medical psychiatry. To have what has been a disturbing, perplexing and disabling state of mind understood as a 'treatable illness' can be immensely reassuring and help some people regain their mental and social functioning. But what is it in the orthodox psychiatric intervention that is therapeutic, given that the efficacy of neuroleptic medication – the *raison d'être* of medical psychiatry – is open to serious challenge (Mosher 2003; Ross & Read 2004). The medicalisation of distress and crises comes at some cost. Firstly, there is the likelihood of long-term medication with all its attendant problems and, secondly, there is the deleterious effect of being labelled for life. But of more significance than this is the fact that it diminishes the opportunity inherent in all crises to learn, grow and change.

· · · · · · · · · · ·

One thing is clear, life is suffering. Although we may like to think of periods of turmoil as aberrations, every human being's life is composed of an emotional ebb and flow in response to the vagaries of existence. Loss and trauma in various guises are the inevitable trials we face as life unfolds. At times the pressures of existence can be so overwhelming that they can hardly be borne and they may then manifest themselves in an array of distressed and disturbed behaviour. Just as our lived experience has both a commonality and uniqueness, so too our troubled states of mind reveal themselves in both common and individual ways. Attempts to classify the turbulent psyche into discrete, reliable, diagnostic categories ultimately fail, as they cannot allow for personal idiosyncrasy and cultural differences. Nor do they account for the frequency with which 'pathological' symptoms occur in the well population.

The boundary between sanity and madness cannot be finely drawn. Bentall (2003) argues that the time has come to abandon the classification of psychiatric disorder – a paradigm that in his view has little scientific merit – and instead to try to understand and explain the *complaints* that people seek help with. It is reasonable to postulate a bell-shaped distribution of wellbeing in the general population, with high levels of wellbeing at one end of the continuum and high levels of distress and disturbance at the other (Fig. 2.1). Where we are at any given moment in our lives on this spectrum of human experience will be determined by the interaction of a complex number of variables. Eastern philosophies equate wellbeing with harmony – a state of grace that flows from experiencing a fundamental 'togetherness' in our inner and outer worlds. If we find ourselves in a discordant or separated state, separated from parts of ourselves, from our social world, from our spiritual heritage, from the biosphere that sustains us, how can we possibly hope to achieve a state of wellbeing?

The theory of distress and disorder that has gained most credibility over the past two decades is the vulnerability–stress model (Zubin & Spring 1977). Unfortunately this model has been hijacked by biomedical psychiatry to advance the theory that it is a genetic-based dysfunction of neurotransmission that is the dominant cause of vulnerability. This narrows down what was intended as a broad focus on the aetiology of troubled states of mind. In its original conception the model postulated that vulnerability to psychological overwhelm could be acquired as a consequence of early psychosocial experiences including trauma and family dysfunction. Bentall, in his insightful book *Madness Explained* (2003), redraws this broader picture of influences which increase our susceptibility to breakdown under stress. Drawing on family studies of insecure attachment, communication deviance and high expressed emotion as a prelude to

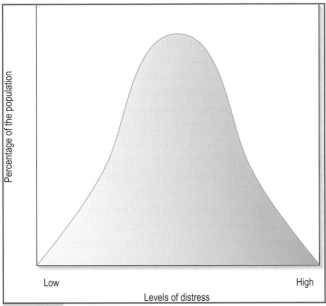

Figure 2.1 ● Levels of distress in the general population. Studies estimate that between 10% and 25% of the population of the UK present with mental health problems annually. Within this figure 2–4% will have severe and disabling levels of distress (Sainsbury Centre for Mental Health 1998).

psychological disturbance in adult life he concludes that there is good evidence that adverse family relationships and interactional patterns increase the risk of the developing child eventually becoming psychotic.

Morrison and colleagues (2003), in a review of the research and theoretical literature, suggest that a significant proportion of psychotic disorders arise in response to trauma. As Read (2004) points out, we should not be surprised that sexual abuse, violence, neglect or parental loss in childhood, often exacerbated by further trauma in adult life, are significant in the aetiology of severe mental health problems, just as they are in that of less disabling manifestations of distress. Furthermore, there is commonly an association between the themes of unusual thoughts and the content of voices – usually regarded as a hallmark of a severe psychological disturbance – and the nature of the traumatic experience. I am reminded of a young man of my acquaintance with a history of depression and voice hearing and an anxious, withdrawn lifestyle, who attributed these complaints to a sexual assault when he was four. He claimed never to have felt safe after the incident and even in adult life was convinced that his assailant was 'out there watching and waiting'. His voices, which were constant companions, were boisterous and gregarious and seemed to represent what was missing from his way of being in the world. He explained them tellingly as the voices of 'youngsters who had never had a life' and were intent on living vicariously through him. Unsurprisingly the voices were often critical of his inert, solitary lifestyle.

The exclusive research focus on genetic and biochemical factors in recent years has deflected attention away from one of the most consistent aetiological

19

features of disabling distress, namely the social dimension of experience. Substantial evidence exists to connect poverty, ethnicity and gender causally to disabling distress. Poverty is a reality that colours the lives of many people. Even in societies where the population generally has enough to eat and somewhere to live, deprivation and disadvantage exist and add significantly to the trials of life. It is an undeniable fact that, as with physical disease, psychological distress is more prevalent in poorer communities than in more affluent ones. Recent studies of poverty confirm earlier findings and consistently point to a causal link between urban deprivation and psychosis (Rushing & Ortega 1979). Impoverishment is demeaning and disempowering. It lowers self-esteem, reduces access to resources that sustain emotional wellbeing and exposes people to uncongenial living conditions, higher levels of crime and antisocial behaviour. Read (2004) points to a circle of oppression that operates when people enter the psychiatric system. The social conditions of their lives are seldom adequately addressed and the poor are more likely than the affluent middle class to be hospitalised and labelled psychotic. This simply serves to further disempower them, lower their self-esteem, diminish employment prospects and distance their friends and loved ones. He concludes: 'It is profoundly depressing that when the poor and the powerless crack under the strain, experts step in to explain that there is something wrong with their brains and condemn them with their labels, drugs and electricity to even greater depths of powerlessness, hopelessness and loneliness' (p. 168).

The dominant discourse on severe distress in our culture is an ethnocentric Western view that conceptualises it as a dysfunctional state located within the individual. So dominant is this illness hypothesis that it has achieved the status of a truth and provides the authoritative basis for professional expert-led care and treatment. While for many individuals this conception of distress as an illness to be treated by health-care professionals may be relevant and acceptable, it is often inappropriate to people whose beliefs are rooted in non-Western cultures. Furthermore racial stereotyping, cultural insensitivity and oppressive practice within the mental health system remain a common experience of people of Afro-Caribbean, African and Asian extraction in Britain and understandably increase their reluctance to seek help from mental health services (Fernando 1995; Bhugra & Bahl 1999).

It does not require a huge stretch of the imagination to see that some troubled states of mind may be culture-bound and that some distress experiences among ethnic minorities are related to the covert everyday racism that is endemic in Britain despite half a century of multiculturalism. A literature review by Sharpley et al (2001) highlights low self-esteem, brought about by social disadvantage and racism, as a key factor in the high incidence of psychosis among Afro-Caribbean people in England. Nor is it difficult to understand the cultural conflicts faced by the children of migrant families who have grown up in Britain and feel both the pull of Western values and the tug of family traditions and beliefs. But as Fernando points out, it would be a mistake to regard any culture as a fossilised entity; it should be seen more as an emergent process that is influenced by the social and family context as much as tradition. In understanding distress we need to be sensitive to the unique experience of the individual and their family as much as to that person's cultural heritage.

It seems extraordinary that after 50 years of feminism we should still be so insensitive to the mental health needs of women. Anxiety and depression are twice as common in women as in men – a fact which points directly to the social experience of women. In a review of research, the Department of Health (2002a) found that women are more likely than men to live in poverty, to be unemployed or to be in low paid jobs. They experience higher levels of social isolation, particularly as lone parents, and are at much greater risk than men of domestic violence, abuse and sexual violence, factors which contribute significantly to mental health problems. Yet 'psychiatry on the whole demonstrates limited understanding of the social impact of poverty, sexism, racism, parenting issues, sexual abuse and violence in women's lives. All account for much mental distress, but a sticking plaster approach never addresses the issues, so distress just recurs' (cited in *Women's Mental Health*, Department of Health 2002a, p. 23).

At the heart of every troubled state of mind is anxiety, and how we deal with that fearfulness determines the characteristics and course of our distress. Anxiety is of course a psychobiological survival mechanism that has evolved to initiate the fight, flight and freeze responses to clear and present danger. In the 21st century only rarely do we encounter a direct and obvious threat to our physical survival – at least in the developed countries of the world. But threats to our psychological survival surround us all the time and we need to be much more reflective and reflexive than our ancestors to negotiate modern life. The threat that we face is to our personhood. Our task in life is the unfolding of our potential as human beings and integrating those emerging facets of self into a harmonious whole. Many things can happen to us that disrupt this process and cause disharmony and disintegration, particularly if the emergent self is not strongly rooted in self-acceptance and self-esteem. The more internally regulated our sense of self-worth is, the more sustained our growth and development as a person will be. If we have not been able to internalise sufficient self-regard from secure and loving attachments to our caregivers in our formative years, then our sense of self-worth will be too dependent on external approbation and on acquiring the outward symbols of success. We will be more vulnerable to rejection, disappointment, loss and failure. We will seek the regard of others in compliant behaviour rather than being authentically who we are. Wholeness means that we acknowledge in ourselves not only all that is virtuous but our failings as well, for not to acknowledge our shadow would mean that our way of being in the world was not fully and authentically human.

The longer medical perspectives dominate the thinking about a person's troubled state of mind, the more the origins of that distress become obscured. There can be little doubt that the most severe mental health problems have their origins not only in life's major traumas but also in what Anthony Trollope called the small, everyday 'lacerations of the spirit'. As we shall see in the next chapter, 'Roads to recovery', the process of becoming a patient may add to this traumatisation. The person who finds her- or himself on the point of disintegration may have had little opportunity to grow and flourish in the context of nurturing formative relationships. They may have always felt a profound and often painful perplexity and insecurity about themselves, their experience and how to be in the world – what R.D. Laing spoke of as *ontological insecurity.* Within the psychiatric system that perplexity and insecurity can unwittingly be compounded by the mystification of diagnosis and the care and treatment process. What people need in the midst of their threatening confusion is to feel safe and grounded and to begin to make some sense of their experience. It must seem utterly bewildering to be told that what seems most real about your experience is an illness, that you need to be admitted to hospital and to take medication. No wonder there is protest! In the end people submit, take their drugs, become somnambulists, keep quiet about their experiences and eventually get discharged. Subsequently and consequently they enter a dispiriting and disempowering cycle of relapses. How much more sense it makes to recognise that what we are witnessing in people's struggles is a transition; a transition in which they are being called to a way of being that is more compatible with harmony and health. What is needed is a recovery environment that nurtures and supports a return to sanity. People need around them others who will be companions on a journey of discovery and recovery; a journey in which the meaning in their distress experiences are uncovered; in which a stronger sense of self emerges; through which a life that has meaning and value is recovered.

Is it possible to see psychological suffering as a gift and not an affliction? A gift which, if we can receive it, allows us to access the richness of our true being, to discard the pretensions of the ego and become more fully ourselves? Can our capacity to experience deep sorrow or exalted excitement, to hear voices or think unusual thoughts make us more human – travellers in the outer reaches of the human psyche? Can we return from such explorations with a deeper and more profound understanding of ourselves, of what it means to be human, an understanding which will shape our way of being in the world? Kay Redfield Jamison, Professor of Psychiatry at the Johns Hopkins University School of Medicine, has written in a profound and illuminating way about her own experience of bipolar disorder. In the epilogue to her memoir she eloquently describes the gift of suffering:

> *I honestly believe that as the result of it I have felt more things, more deeply; had more experiences, more intensely; loved more, and been more loved; laughed more often for having cried more often; appreciated more the springs, for all the winters; worn death 'as close as dungarees', appreciated it – and life more; seen the finest and the most terrible in people, and slowly learnt the values of caring, loyalty and seeing things through ...*

> *Even when I have been at my most psychotic – delusional, hallucinating, frenzied – I have been aware of finding new corners of my mind and heart. Some of those corners were incredible and beautiful and took my breath away and made me feel as if I could die right then and the images would sustain me. Some of them were grotesque and ugly and I never wanted to know they were there or to see them again. But always there were those new corners – and when feeling my*

normal self, beholden for that self to medicine and love – I cannot imagine becoming jaded to life, because I know those limitless corners, with their limitless views. (Jamison 1993)

Many people who have experienced extreme and incapacitating distress would not see it as an adversity or an illness to be treated and alleviated, despite the suffering involved. They would instead see it as part of who they are, part of the panoply of human experience from which a stronger, more compassionate, harmonious and creative self can emerge. Because medical psychiatry tends to stifle this process by reducing distress and disturbance in the psyche to a disorder to be treated, many survivors of the psychiatric system have not recognised and seized the opportunity to develop and grow until they have regained some sovereignty over their lives and have been able to answer the call to begin the recovery journey.

Voices of experience – a personal reflection on recovery

Janet Russell

In a fit of introspection, on turning 60, I came to the not very original conclusion that I am the sum of all that has happened in my life. Likewise, the child that I had been inevitably grew into the mute, isolated, overweight woman who sat, drugged and dribbling, day after day, in the corner of a ward in our local psychiatric hospital. Thirteen years ago, I was locked into this existence and there seemed to be no door into the outside world.

I was an only child, a strange, solitary girl, who would prefer to have my nose in a book or be inventing stories and companions in my head to risking confrontation with real people. I had friends, but could really manage only one at a time. I was an academic high-flyer, mainly because I spent most of my youth swotting. I knew that I was different, unattractive and unlovable, and the only way I could shine was to do well at school. I had to be top; second was not good enough.

I trained to be a teacher. Shortly after qualifying, I married a fellow student. I knew that this was a mistake, since I was aware that he was unstable, cruel and self-centred, but I married him out of gratitude and because I knew that nobody else would want me. His constant physical and emotional violence destroyed what tiny amount of self-esteem I had. The 'blues' of my youth descended into deep depression. Eventually, during my second admission to hospital, he decided that I had nothing more to offer and abandoned me. This seemed to me totally justified, deserved and predictable.

I had left teaching by this time, unable to cope with the pressure, and obtained a well-paid, soul-destroying job in the civil service. I picked up the threads of my life alone. Soon, however, I realised that the milkman was poisoning my milk and that there was a man constantly standing opposite my house, watching my every move. Eventually, I was sectioned and, for the next seven years, spent more time in hospital than at home. Inevitably, I lost my job. From being an intelligent pro-fessional woman, I felt that I was now nothing. The few acquaintances that I had fell away, and I was totally isolated. My family was supportive but bewildered and helpless.

During the 1970s, I was given large doses of drugs, in every imaginable combin-ation. I felt barely conscious for most of the time. Three times a week I was shipped off to the women's dormitory, where dozens were subjected to ECT. At the weekly ward conference, I was surrounded by mental health workers and professionals, all with much to say about my progress – or lack of it. I would be talked over, but never addressed or allowed to open my mouth. Typically, the consultant would bark an enquiry as to whether I was improving. On being told that I was not, he would imme-diately snap back, 'Give her another six (or 12, or 20) shots of ECT'. But ECT made my depression deeper and me less able to think or function.

Towards the end of that decade, several personal traumas occurred within a matter of weeks. I was so befuddled with drugs that I was unable to think things through. Hospital staff were not trained to talk to patients or even accept their humanity. One afternoon, I roused myself from my stupor sufficiently to smash a very large window in the dining area. I soon found myself locked in a dark, shuttered room, totally empty except for a mattress, a blanket and a bedpan. I am told that I was there until the following morning. That night, voices came to shout at me about my wickedness, worthlessness, filth, and malign effect upon the world.

Twenty-seven years later, these two voices are still with me. They are there when I wake in the morning and they are there when I go to sleep at night. It is hard to explain how it felt that first night that they arrived. I was scared, alone, desperate, cold and uncomfortable. There was no way that anyone could have spoken to me from outside that room. I was too drugged to think of any rational explanation for their presence. They were – and are – totally real. That they were telling me things that I already knew about myself made them all the more powerful and completely believable. They told me the world would become infected, and eventually destroyed, if I did not kill myself. By the time that the door was opened in the morning, I was gibbering with terror. The voices forbade me to tell anyone about them and I kept them a secret for nearly 10 years.

In 1980, I discharged myself from hospital. For the next seven years, I fought my way back to some sort of normality. I was liberated from medication, and so able to think straight again. I got various low paid jobs before getting work with more responsibility and challenge, and pleasant workmates. I made a few friends. I became deeply involved in my church and soon became leader of a number of organisations, especially with young people. They were difficult times but the new friendships, the sense of worth and achievement and my increasing Christian faith enabled me to continue.

My success, however, was my downfall. I took on more and more and eventually became exhausted and burned out. I was good at my job but lost my confidence, could not cope and survived only because workmates were covering for me. The voices were constantly shouting, loud and clear. I was becoming terrified of what would happen if I did not comply with their orders. Soon, I was again sectioned and it seemed as if the progress of the previous years had evaporated.

I spent almost the whole of the next four and a half years in hospital. During that time, I lost my job and most of my friends drifted away. The treatment offered me was precisely the same as before – medication. I was given ever increasing doses of neuroleptics, none of which had any effect at all on the voices. The medication only made me lethargic, overweight and unable to think. I just sat in a bay window, saying and doing nothing other than listening to the threats and taunts of the voices. My 'care' was taken over by another consultant, who was determined to 'sort me out', at any cost. I was subjected to another course of ECT and to several 'unusual' treatments, including abreaction and sleep deprivation. I did not consent to, nor was I told the purpose of, being kept awake for 72 hours, but the only apparent result was that the volume and virulence of the voices escalated considerably. In addition, long-term use of high doses of neuroleptics resulted in my developing tardive dyskinesia. I was dribbling; I shook so much that I often could not drink from a cup; I was shuffling like a pensioner; I was grimacing to the extent that my mother was embarrassed to take me out. But none of these facts were of any concern to anyone but me, and I was a non-person. The thing I longed for most was to be able to talk to someone about how I felt. However, whenever I tried to discuss the voices with staff members, I was told that 'We don't talk about things that aren't there. When you stop talking nonsense, we'll come back.'

Eventually, I was transferred to another consultant who, I think out of desperation, agreed to my coming off all medication. I was sent to the rehabilitation unit and, over seven months, the tablets were withdrawn. After a couple of months, I began to feel alive again. Gradually, I began noticing the world around me. It was like being reborn. I was able to do my own cooking, to dabble with computers, to take up carpentry. I was once more a person. On 15 June 1993, I was discharged from hospital and began a new life.

Life wasn't easy. Sometimes the voices were so intense that I felt I had to comply with them. I worked with an art therapist for several years, who was the first person who listened to me. The single most helpful thing in my rehabilitation was the relationship I had with my key worker at an activities centre I attended. He expressed interest in the voice hearing experience and, together, we embarked on a voyage of discovery that involved us in contact with the Hearing Voices Network, going to conferences and workshops, and hour upon hour of discussion. I explored every aspect of the voices – their sex, ages, personalities, what angered or pleased them, when they were most insistent. I became so familiar with them that they seemed less mysterious and threatening. I found devices to put them to the back of my mind so that they were less intrusive. I began to feel more in control and less at their mercy. It was a relief to have the voices taken seriously and acknowledged as a reality. My key worker gave me unlimited time, attention and non-judgmental support. I had another terrifying breakdown in 1997 and he spent hours, just sitting in my living room and sharing the experience of the voices attacking me. His support continues, on a different level, to this day. I was also very blessed to have almost three years of psychotherapy with an amazing psychologist who, almost imperceptibly, helped me to understand myself and even to love myself a bit.

I took up creative writing, something I had always dabbled in, and wrote a lot of poetry. I feel perversely thankful that I was able to 'touch the bottom' of myself, in a way few people can. The poems were very vivid and full of strange images and pain. Their literary value was limited but writing them was very therapeutic and helped me to understand myself. I joined a class and began to do 'proper' writing. It was much better crafted but in the comparative tranquillity of recent years I have never been able to recapture the intensity of those early poems. Eventually I gained a first class university diploma in creative writing – a treasured qualification.

Shortly after leaving hospital, with help from the Shaw Trust, I was able to get a part-time job at the local council, which I held for six years. After this, I worked for four years as a support worker with a voluntary sector mental health community support team. This was immensely rewarding, if sometimes harrowing, and something I felt uniquely qualified to do. I left only recently to care for my elderly, sick parents, something that I am so thankful to be able to do and which I did not think I would ever be able to do. The opportunity to demonstrate that I could work consistently and effectively, to study at university level and write successfully, raised my self-esteem considerably. I now feel much more in control of my own life. Although I am vulnerable, my vulnerability gives a strange strength and invincibility.

I see now that, had I been given talking therapy and support when I first became 'ill' in 1969, instead of being destroyed by endless drugs, I would have had a different life. Good relationships and personal support are vital. I know now that my long-held belief that I was at the mercy of the voices is not true. They are still very 'real' and often problematic; I would not claim to be 'cured' or dispute the fact that I may have further episodes of psychosis. But I can see that the voices are a manifestation of my own perception of myself, and that I do not have to follow their instructions.

When, in 2000, I was told by a consultant psychiatrist that I had never been ill because if I had been I could not have recovered to the extent that I have, I was hurt and angry. His calling my voices 'pseudo voices' is something I cannot accept. Seen from his viewpoint it has taken the medical profession 31 years, six consultants and enough drugs to knock out the population of London to come to the conclusion that there was nothing wrong with me! I can rejoice that my recovery – won by my own efforts and the love of friends – is sufficient to explain, if not justify, this last diagnosis!

Roads to recovery

3

You enter the forest at the darkest part, where there is no path. . . The idea is to find your own pathway to bliss.

Joseph Campbell

Introduction

Western psychiatry has tended to hold an attitude of therapeutic pessimism about the impact of severe mental health problems on the lives of people seeking help. The prognosis for the majority has been the likelihood of further relapses and some inevitable deterioration in mental and social functioning. Long-term adherence to antipsychotic medication has been seen as offering the best chance of maintaining a symptom-free life and a reasonable level of social functioning. It is still rare for people to be considered recovered, even if they have been symptom-free for many years. 'In remission' is the preferred explanation. This cautious view of recovery has been challenged over the past decade by the more optimistic outcomes of longitudinal studies which indicate the possibility of a full recovery or significant improvement for up to two-thirds of people whose psychotic experiences have resulted in a psychiatric diagnosis (Harrison et al 2001). Even this figure may be seen as unduly conservative, since studies are commonly based on exacting, measurable recovery criteria such as those proposed by Liberman et al (2002), namely the absence of symptoms for two consecutive years, a socially inclusive lifestyle, including some employment activity, and evidence of sustained independent living. These criteria do not encompass an individual's subjective experience of wellbeing and recovery – recovery of a meaningful and fulfilling life despite, in some cases, the continuation of symptoms and episodic distress (Davidson 2003). A further challenge to the prevailing therapeutic pessimism has come from the published recovery testimonies of mental health system consumers and survivors (Barker et al 1999; Read & Reynolds 2000; Barker & Buchanan-Barker 2004). The convergent view to be drawn from these autobiographical reflections is that recovery is a process of accepting and transcending a vulnerability to overwhelming psychological distress and dysfunction in the pursuit of whatever life goals and aspirations an individual sets for him- or herself.

The growing empirical and experiential evidence that clinical and social recovery from severe mental health problems is not only possible but probable has, over the past decade, provided the guiding vision for the reorientation of mental health services in America (Anthony 1993) and more recently in Britain (Department of Health 2001). If this reconfiguration of services is to be more than mere re-branding, our task as mental health professionals is to ensure that our practice is rooted in a humanistic, person-centred philosophy and exemplifies competencies conducive to recovery (Box 3.1):

Box 3.1

Characteristics of a recovery culture

- Acknowledge people as experts in their own experience
- Recognise and support the personal resourcefulness of individuals
- Recognise that recovery is a unique process and that there are many roads to the well-lived life
- Recognise the importance of social inclusion and full citizenship in recovery and seek to promote it
- Embrace the diversity of views on the nature of psychological distress
- Enable people to discover meaning in their experience of distress that is personally relevant
- Sustain and communicate the belief in the potential of people to grow and change in life-enhancing ways
- Recognise the positive elements in a person's vulnerability, and that breakdown can lead to breakthrough
- Accept setbacks as an inevitable part of the recovery journey and see them as opportunities for fresh insights, growth and change
- Recognise that recovering from the social consequences of severe, enduring psychological distress and psychiatric diagnosis can be more difficult than re-covering from the mental health problem itself
- See our role as mental health professionals in the recovery process as collaborative and facilitative rather than authoritative
- Affirm strengths, skills, qualities and abilities rather than maintain an imbalanced focus on deficits
- Accept that people can recover without professional help
- Respect the rights of individuals to self-determination and choice
- Understand the importance of the family system and personal support networks in the recovery process
- Maintain a culturally sensitive approach to working with people in their recovery process
- Support the role of the user/survivor movement in the development and valid-ation of training and the reconfiguration and auditing of the service provision

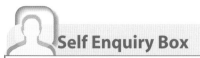

Self Enquiry Box

You may find it useful to reflect on your current practice in relation to the individual recovery competencies listed above and rate yourself using the scale below. This might be a useful focus for peer group supervision, individual supervision or a team review of practice. With some minor adaptation it could be used as a basis for a consumer audit of a recovery service. Alternatively, rate yourself on the competencies and ask your clients to give you feedback. Ask yourself what specifically needs to change in the thinking/feeling/behavioural dimension of your practice for you to more fully embrace a particular competency.

5. I always hold and express this attitude in my practice

4. I mostly hold and express this attitude in my practice

3. I sometimes hold and express this attitude in my practice

2. I occasionally hold and express this attitude in my practice

1. I do not subscribe to and express this attitude in my practice

A definition of what recovery means needs to be our starting point. Some people define their emergence from a deeply troubled state of mind simply as 'regaining self-confidence and control over my life'. Others recognise that recovery has involved personal growth: 'I accept and value myself a lot more and because of that I'm a happier person'. More prosaically, Roe et al (2004) describe recovery as a process of self-discovery, renewal and transformation. It can be a lengthy, painful and difficult process but one that leads to the emergence of a new sense of self, one that is more vital and meaningful, and to the enrichment of one's connections with others. Similarly Roberts & Wolfson (2004) highlight the growing interest in a radical redefinition of recovery 'as a process of personal discovery, of how to live (and live well) with enduring symptoms and vulnerabilities'.

As we saw in the introduction to this chapter, conventional recovery research has tended to measure recovery according to a level of social functioning and the control or absence of symptoms (social and clinical recovery), with little thought given to the personal subjective experience of the people involved or the quality of their lives. Many people who experience overwhelming, troubled states of mind would not see the disappearance of symptoms such as voice hearing as being a hallmark of recovery. They may be living satisfying, contributing lives while still experiencing voices, cognitive difficulties or significant mood swings. What is important and what distinguishes this group from those still troubled, and for whom life has remained restricted, is that the former group has been able to integrate their experience of psychological turmoil into an essentially positive identity. This has largely come about because they have been able to attribute personal meaning to their complaints and have found ways of overcoming or minimising these, rather than their complaints continuing to overwhelm and dominate their lives. This has allowed them to actualise more of their potential, utilise their strengths, pursue their dreams and reclaim a life for themselves – a life with the same measure of joys and satisfactions to which we all aspire.

Taken outside the context of medical psychiatry, recovery is not a particularly helpful term for what is essentially a process of growth and change. Given enabling circumstances, we are all in a state of becoming – always redefining ourselves and realising our innate potential as human beings in response to the flow of life experience. Such a process is not a destination but an ongoing journey. Few of us ever fully become what Rogers (1961) termed a 'fully functioning person', free of defensiveness, open and responsive to life's experience.

Rogers' conception of the change process was of an action tendency that manifests itself as *stasis* at one end of the continuum and *fluidity* at the other (Fig. 3.1). The more our emotional equilibrium is disturbed, the more the social fabric of our lives is disrupted, the more our dreams and hopes are destroyed, then the more profound the required change can be (Roe et al 2004). But it is often the case that when people have been subjected to a bewildering and overwhelming period of distress they become stuck (*in stasis*), unable to grow and change and live life within a restricting zone of safety. Previous conceptions of self and reality have changed, the familiar matrix of life has been shaken up in the turbulent mind and, as a consequence, it is difficult to know how to be in the world.

The focus of recovery work is on enabling people to free themselves from this developmental stasis and emerge from a zone of safety. Stepping out from this static way of being requires an act of courage, of will, of hopefulness. It requires people to face the challenges, opportunities and responsibilities of life. It requires people to confront the emotional legacies of past traumas, to be able to reconfigure their sense of self, one that incorporates the past but is not weakened by it. In addition to this there may be the numbing effect of continuing medication, the loss of personhood in the process of becoming a psychiatric patient and the impoverishment of social exclusion to contend with. All of this is hard work. Small wonder that many people settle for stasis.

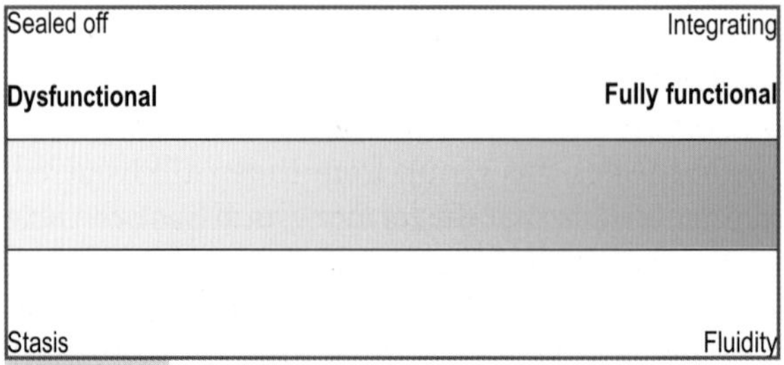

Sealed off	Integrating
Dysfunctional	**Fully functional**
Stasis	Fluidity

Figure 3.1 The change continuum.

The hero's journey

It is often helpful to explore a complex process with the aid of a metaphor. I have found it useful to think about the often lengthy and convoluted process of recovery as a journey and in particular *a hero's (and heroine's) journey*. The mythology of the hero's journey is embedded in human history and like all myths has something profound to say about the nature of human existence and how to live our lives. The hero's journey portrays an individual setting out on a quest, confronting many challenges and ultimately returning home changed by the experience. At the heart of all myths is a message that reveals something of the mystery of human existence and experience. Contained within the mythic story is the essence of what it is to be human. It is about suffering and redemption; alienation and connectedness; heartlessness and love; meaning and confusion; suffering and joy; death and rebirth. We find the hero's journey in the classical Greek epic tale *The Odyssey* and in a contemporary counterpart, *The Lord of the Rings*. We see it personified in modern times by leaders of the civil rights and anti-apartheid movements, in the acts of sporting legends, in humanitarian endeavours, and in great scientific or artistic achievement, all of which come out of belief, commitment and struggle. All human life can be seen as a hero's journey in which the quest is to be more fully alive, to find a way of being in which we experience 'the rapture of life' (Campbell 1993). In the classical hero's journey – as in the recovery journey – there are many stages: the call; the mentor; the threshold; the way; the return.

The call

Quest: to recognise the imperative nature of the call and to answer yes to life

There is a point at which life begins to feel untenable. We are prompted by increasing levels of distress to seek a resolution; to seek a different, less anguished way of being in the world. That prompting may take the form of increasingly disturbing, extraordinary states of consciousness; or of overwhelming, troubled sadness, paralysing anxieties, dangerous and disfiguring self-harm, or destructive addictions. Often we do not recognise these manifestations of distress for what they are, signs of disharmony in our inner and outer worlds. Dis-ease in mind or body, or both, is always a message from the unconscious, alerting us to a loss of equilibrium in our lives. This lack of awareness is reinforced by pathologising symptoms of distress, which further dislocates them from their true source and removes the responsibility to act; a process that encourages passivity, hopelessness and victimhood. The use of neuroleptic drugs may contribute further to this disabling process by suppressing emotional tensions that can be the mainspring of motivation to engage in recovery work. Schiff (2004), in a personal reflection and analysis of her recovery from mental illness, identifies the role of emotional pain as an initiator of her recovery journey, stating that 'settling into a state of numbness' would have blocked her healing process. After a time the original source of the distress becomes obscure and the task of making the connections that lead to meaning and insight becomes more difficult.

Often the call generates its own fearfulness. To rescue one's life from the grip of inner demons and a marginalised existence can seem an impossible quest. It can be difficult to transcend the state of dispiritedness that may have settled over an individual's life and hard to overcome a prevailing sense of hopelessness and helplessness sufficiently to take the risk of striking out in the direction of a more fulfilling way of being and living. It may be easier to stay sealed off in the comfort zone of a life circumscribed by mental illness.

Some people are able to adopt an *integrating* recovery style while others adopt a *sealing over* coping strategy in response to troubled and distressed states of mind (see Fig. 3.1). Tait et al (2003), in their study of engagement patterns, describe *sealing over* as characterised by a lack of curiosity about the distress experience and an avoidance of any active involvement in discovering more functional coping strategies. Sealing over, as a defence against the threat to identity and self-esteem posed by the experience of a severe psychological crisis, leads to dis-engagement or passive engagement with services and militates against recovery (Birchwood et al 2000). There are likely to be numerous psychosocial factors at work in determining the recovery style of individuals, such as the habitual crisis response patterns learned in a person's family of origin. Despite this seemingly entrenched recovery style, it is possible to emerge from a sealed-over way of coping over time, given appropriate psychological support (see Chapter 8, 'Recovery relationships'). Indicators that a person is becoming less defensive are a greater willingness to engage in discussions about problems in living; the meaning of distress symptoms and ways of managing them; appearing less sunk in their distress or occupied with displacing their distress; and having more energy for living.

In the recovery journey there may be many starts and many retreats before the call is answered with a sustained 'yes' to a life that offers more.

Empowerment in answering the call

Responding positively to the call both requires and engenders a sense of personal empowerment. If we no longer feel in control of our lives it is difficult to believe we have the capability to change anything. Personal power is that sense of autonomy and self-efficacy that enables us to become responsible and resource-ful individuals, able to manage and influence the direction of our unfolding lives. Coleman (1999) puts it this way:

> I am one of those who hold to the idea that personal recovery has at its very heart the reclamation of personal power. In order for the recovery journey to be success-ful I believe it is important to deconstruct the power of the psychiatric system and to reconstruct power as a personal commodity. (p. 48)

Personal power is a dimension of the self that ebbs and flows in response to psychosocial and political influences throughout life. The power invested in social roles is particularly evident in the power imbalance of professional helping relationships, an issue that has been the subject of a continuing debate over the past 20 years. Campbell (2000), writing of his own encounters with the mental health care system, cites the experience of being invalidated as a 'cognisant, competent, creative person, as a consequence of being diagnosed mentally ill' as being an insidious force that diminishes and disempowers people. There is now great emphasis on the need for partnership and collaborative working relationships between clients and mental health professionals and managing this dynamic in relationships is a key factor in recovery. The way power is held and used varies along a continuum from being authoritative at one end to facilitative at the other. The longer someone is subjected to authoritative relationships, the more personal power is surrendered, with the individual sliding towards a passive compliant attitude. Conversely, the relationship may become more conflicted as the individual desperately attempts to reassert their diminishing personal power. This latter scenario may express itself in challenging behaviour, non-engagement, non-adherence to care and treatment plans and a rejection of diagnostic formulations, a situation which often results in the use or threatened use of coercive legal power, which is a further demeaning assault on a person's sovereignty, diminishing the control they have over their lives.

The dynamic of disempowerment can be, and often is, more complicated than this. Frequently a poorly developed sense of autonomy predates a person's referral to psychiatric services. It may be a distinguishing feature of an individual's personality and a causative factor in their current level of distress. This established pattern of behaviour is thus likely to readily manifest itself in helping relationships, with the client relinquishing power and rapidly adopting a helpless and dependent role. This needs to be openly acknowledged and worked with as a starting point for encouraging and strengthening the personal agency of the individual and as the basis for meeting dependency needs in more adaptive ways. The flip side of this scenario can be that the professional helper's own denied dependency needs are met by projecting them on to the client and satisfied vicariously. It is a mechanism that imputes to those seeking help a greater degree of vulnerability and fragility than is justified.

Not only do our dependency needs come into play in our caring role but also our need to feel powerful, perhaps to mask a sense of insecurity and powerlessness which we experience for a complexity of reasons, both linked to our personal history and socially constructed. These personal needs and emotional hurts, mostly outside of our awareness, that intrude into the dynamics of helping relationships underlie what Heron (2001) calls contaminated helping – the shadow side of helping. They are an example of why self-awareness and personal development training should be a visible strand of the education of mental health professionals and why supervision is a vital resource in the maintenance of good practice (Watkins 2001).

I am not arguing here that there are never times when a more authoritative caring response is needed. People in the grip of anguish and despair, disturbed and distracted by a perplexing and threatening reality, may need someone to take responsibility for their wellbeing for a time. Even so, responding in directive, prescriptive ways to a person's care needs can usually be done in a consultative way that is respectful of the client's capacity for self-determination, however diminished that might be at a given moment in time.

The prescriptive use of power is one of the most contentious areas of mental health care and a central reason why many system survivors feel a deep mistrust

33

of psychiatry and advocate that real empowerment and recovery can only begin once they have freed themselves from the psychiatric services. This is a damning indictment of a system of care that tries to do the impossible; a system that has invested in it the responsibility of balancing and integrating the dual roles of caring/healing with social control. Sadly it is the controlling power of the psychiatric system, as experienced and witnessed by people using the service, that for many has become the face of psychiatry. It is characterised by the loss of freedom through legally enforced hospitalisation; the coercive or enforced use of neuroleptic drugs; the locked doors of admission units; the use of close observation; the use of physical restraint and seclusion in response to distressed and disturbed behaviour. To be the recipient of such experiences is to be subjected to an assault on the sovereignty of the self that leaves many people feeling subjugated and diminished. This is unlikely to change until the mental health service opens itself fully to the humanitarian gaze of a more compassionate society.

There are too many 'experts' in the psychiatric professions who are all too ready to provide answers to suffering and the problems in living for which people seek help, a stance which increasingly seems to my mind to be an act of deception. If we take the expression of human suffering outside the framework of mental illness, then treatment and cure is clearly an inappropriate aim. In the multi-disciplinary world of the helping professions in recent years, there has been an anxious preoccupation with credibility, status and power. Most disciplines have sought to underpin their position by becoming ever more 'knowledgeable doers' whose practice is evidence based. While there are some laudable elements to this, it appears to me to have been at the cost of a more human and profound approach to helping, a collaborative quest for a shared understanding of suffering and for a less troubled way of being and living. As Thomas & Bracken (2004) note, psychiatry patrols the boundary between reason and unreason. It holds the high ground of reason and professes that unreason is only knowable through the language of reason, which excludes the voice of those persons deemed mentally ill. It disregards the capacity of people for reflection and introspection, to be observers and interpreters of their own subjective world, to travel through an inner landscape shaped by other realities and find meaning there.

Whatever the underlying dynamic, disempowerment is a significant barrier to recovery. Ahern & Fisher (2001), drawing on their recovery research conducted under the auspices of the National Empowerment Centre, identify empowerment as the necessary condition for recovery work to be effective. They argue that the healing of severe emotional distress is more effective in an empowerment culture than in the hierarchical, expert-centred culture of the psychiatric system. An empowerment culture is one in which someone is exposed to recovery relationships that have at their heart a belief in the individual's worth and in their capacity to live through severe distress and to learn and grow from the crisis experience; relationships in which the subjective experience of the person seeking help is validated and where there is a search for meaning that has relevance to the person's lived experience. It is a culture that enables someone to reconstruct a positive identity from one that has been fragmented and supplanted by the overwhelming experience of being deeply disturbed and distressed; one that offers social inclusion and a meaningful role rather than the socially marginalised experience of many mental health service users (Box 3.2).

Box 3.2

Creating an empowerment culture

Some general points:

- Allow more time for people: for listening; for talking; for doing things together
- Normalise helping relationships/develop person-to-person relationships
- Flatten the hierarchical structure
- Avoid mystifying, excluding jargon
- Respect the way people experience their reality
- Respect the expertise of people in knowing what helps
- Avoid pathologising labels and deterministic explanations
- Provide the accessible information needed to be able to make informed choices and ensure it is understood
- Encourage people to take a leading role in their own care planning process
- Help people to recognise they are their own best resource
- Enable people to access resources outside the service provision to meet their needs – such as education/training, complementary therapies or recreational facilities
- Respect people's right to choose
- Practice judicious non-intervention
- Respect people's right to the dignity of risk
- Avoid coercion and threats
- Celebrate people's achievements, successes, strengths and abilities
- Nurture hopefulness
- Help people gain the skills they need to feel more empowered and be more assertive
- Acknowledge the impact of social inequalities and impoverishment on the lives of people using mental health services
- Acknowledge the impact of stigma on the lives of people who use mental health services
- Avoid using mythologising/stereotyping/abusive language to describe people using services; terms like 'attention seeker', 'waster', 'schizo'
- Openly discuss the experiences of compulsory admission, detention, observation, treatment
- Develop an ethos of a caring/healing community to which everyone gives and receives
- Encourage the use of advocacy
- Encourage involvement in service user forums
- Seek consumers' views on the service and encourage user-led research

Self Enquiry Box

Using the rating scale below, you might find it helpful to consider the factors identified in Box 3.2 as significant in creating an empowerment culture and consider the extent to which these are present in your service. This could be the basis for a staff team discussion or useful as part of a collaborative review of a service involving client feedback. Consider how you might develop those factors receiving a low rating in your service culture.

5. This factor is a constant presence of our service

4. This factor is mostly present in our service

3. This factor is sometimes present in our service

2. This factor is occasionally present in our service

1. We do not value or express this factor in our service

The heroes of literature almost always have flaws and failings. Many have deep wounds which bear witness to past hurts such as loss, abuse, rejection, abandonment to which they are driven to find a resolution. Many have a non-heroic persona; they are not the brave and the bold of legend. This makes their journeys all the more courageous and teaches us that everyone can find heroic qualities within themselves.

Grieving the life not lived in answering the call

LaFond (2002) makes the case that significant loss, trauma and deprivation are frequently a consequence of serious mental health problems and healing the emotional wounds inflicted by these loss experiences is a necessary phase of recovery work. Only when the reality of what has happened to us has been acknowledged and a stage of acceptance reached is recovery work possible. Often the continuing denial, sadness and protest associated with enduring distress and disorder make it difficult for people to respond positively to the call to begin the task of reclaiming their lives and rebuilding their identities. As mental health professionals we have not been sufficiently aware and responsive to this loss experience, either failing to recognise the magnitude of the losses involved or tending to pathologise the grief reaction, seeing it as part of the symptomology of a person's primary distress.

For the individual whose life has been disrupted by overwhelming distress and disturbance there can be many losses and traumas. Being given a diagnosis such as schizophrenia can be devastating, as can compulsory hospital admission and detention under the Mental Health Act. Being adrift in a sea of turmoil, cut off from the familiar anchorage of the life one knows can be frightening and regaining one's moorings can be hard to do. Personal and family relationships are strained and sometimes broken, friends are lost or become distant, educational experience is disrupted, career prospects and work opportunities may be diminished. In the psychological sphere of one's life a different reality has settled over once familiar territory, ushered in by unusual thoughts, perceptions and profound mood changes. In some perplexing way life is the same yet different. We are the same – yet not who we were. Within the totality of this experience is an enormous loss, yet a loss which is largely unrecognised by society and indeed by many mental health professionals.

As Andy Dufresne says to his friend and fellow 'lifer' Red in the film *The Shawshank Redemption*, 'You either get busy living or get busy dying'. But we can only get busy living when we have mourned the loss of the life not lived. Grieving goes through stages: overcoming denial and acknowledging loss; facing the sadness, anger, fear and guilt that are an expression of the pain of loss; and ultimately coming to an acceptance of one's vulnerability to distress and of the life not lived (Box 3.3). For many people the recovery journey may be impeded by this unresolved grief. They may feel anger and resentment about the way in which services have intervened in crises. The trauma of compulsory admissions,

---

Box 3.3

The tasks of grieving

Acknowledging the reality of what's happened

- How often does a client talk about living with a mental health problem and the effect it has had on the fabric of his or her life/identity/aspirations and dreams?

Key question: How has your life changed since you first began to experience mental health problems?

Facing the pain of grief

- How often does a client talk about/express feelings connected with losses incurred in having an enduring mental health problem?

Key question: How have these events in your life left you feeling?

Adjusting to a life that has changed

- How accepting is the client of his/her vulnerability to mental health problems?
- How effective are they at integrating what has happened into a positive identity?
- How active is the client in imagining and reconstructing a future for him-/herself?

Key question: When you are on the more solid ground of recovery what will be in place in your life that's not present now?

Emotionally investing in the future

- How easily is the client able to find happiness/pleasure/ satisfaction in her/his newly emerging identity/life?
- How strong is their self-esteem and confidence?

Key question: What are the positives in the way you and your life have changed?

(Adapted from Worden 1991)

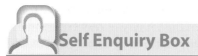

Self Enquiry Box

You may find it useful to reflect on your work with clients who seem to have un-resolved grief issues relating to the impact of their mental health problem on their lives. Use the schema in Box 3.3 as a way of conceptualising where they are in their grieving process. The framework can be used as a basis for dialogue with clients around grief issues. Remember that grieving is not a straightforward linear process and that people vacillate backwards and forwards through the stages of grief. Remember too that there is no time limit on grief – it can take some time to reach a resolution.

enforced treatment and imposed diagnosis can leave a legacy of resentment, fear and distrust. Feelings of bitterness may be present about not being heard and understood by professionals, about the invalidation of subjective experience and the loss of personhood that have often typified the psychiatric process. For some people there may be a pervasive sense of guilt; a sense that they have in some way brought this misfortune on themselves; that they have been 'weak minded' and 'weak willed'; that they have caused disruption and unhappiness in the social sphere of their lives. Such self-recrimination can cloud a person's emotional life. There can be a sense of injustice and sadness about the psychological turmoil which has erupted into their life and which has had such a destructive effect on the fabric of their existence, their career, their relationships, and robbed them of their dreams and aspirations.

The grief scenario may often be quite complicated. One service user of my acquaintance, who has a long history of engagement (and disengagement) with mental health services, is an example of someone whose unresolved grief has made it difficult for him to answer the call to begin his recovery journey. He is a man who experiences wild fluctuations in mood and paranoid hostility. His conversation reveals much unresolved grief over being abandoned by his parents as a child; over the loss of his Caribbean heritage, having grown up in predominantly white British foster homes; over the loss of 'educational opportunities' having inappropriately been sent to a special school for pupils with learning difficulties. The theme of loss has followed him into adult life in the form of a loss of opportunity 'to be someone' with a 'normal life' – to have a relationship, a job, a car, a home. That this has not happened he attributes to his psychiatric history, which has included numerous admissions, often enforced under the Mental Health Act. The betrayals and deprivations of the past, the loss of his right – the birthright of all children – to be a loved and lovable child, find echoes in the present in the form of his marginalised life and 'spoilt' identity. He has never accepted an illness conception of his problems in living, rejecting diagnoses such as schizoaffective disorder and paranoid psychosis and instead seeing his problems as an emotional legacy of the multiple losses and traumas that have dogged him through much of his life.

I am well acquainted with grief. In June 2000 my son took his own life. It has taken me six years to remove his last address and telephone number from my address book – a small thing, yet another painful reality check, confirming that he no longer has a physical presence in the world. Such is the subtle persistence of denial and the enduring power of attachment.

My journey through grief has involved enormous pain. In the early stages I drifted through the days like a somnambulist; days punctuated by paroxysms of anguish. At times I did not recognise myself in the cathartic expression of my grief; it sounded so primal. Guilt has been the hardest part of grieving. That I should have recognised the perilous nature of his emotional suffering and kept him safe has continued to be a tormenting thought.

Suicide is an act that threatens to destroy much more than that person's life. It leaves behind a legacy of bitterness at what can be seen as a revengeful act. The enduring sadness can have a corrosive effect that takes the gleam out of life. A mean spirited resentment towards the seemingly blessed nature of other people's lives can blunt your capacity to share in others' joy. An impotent anger, directed at the universal life force that seems to desert many young men and women each year with such tragic consequences, can eat away at your capacity to celebrate life. All of this has to be worked through to find acceptance and peace of mind. It has to be faced and re-evaluated so that one can live with the reality of what has happened. Initially this does not seem possible; the raw awfulness of it is too much to bear.

With suicide you are always left with the question 'Why?' Living with not knowing is difficult. The reasons lie in the complexity of that unique life and are essentially unknowable. Albert Camus, in his essay on suicide, talks about confronting the absurdity of life; he argues that our ultimate task is to overcome a sense of futility through finding a meaning for living, a meaning that draws us on into life (Camus 1955). Although it remains perplexing for those of us who are left to ponder why, we have to accept that in the last analysis, that good enough reason to live crucially remains elusive or is eclipsed in the minds of those who take their own lives.

It is these emotional issues, the byways of grief alluded to above, that the families and friends of people who disappear into a chaotic world of 'madness' often struggle to deal with. For those who succumb to troubled states of mind it is finding a good enough reason to begin rebuilding one's life in the wasteland created by enduring psychological turmoil that is the seed of recovery.

Risk-taking in answering the call

We cannot exclude risk from life – risk is inherent in the quest for a more fulfilled life. No development or change would be possible if risks were not accepted as a necessary part of living. I would also argue that in the process of safeguarding personal sovereignty people have the *right* to be at risk and to take risks. There will always be some tension between the aspirations of people anxious to move forward in their recovery journeys and mental health workers who might allay their own anxieties by advising a more cautious course of action. This some-times has parental/child overtones when the desire to protect someone from potential harm meets the equally powerful force of the need to live a life of one's own. Such a scenario is played out most vividly in disputes around medica-tion, hospitalisation, a choice of housing or discontinuing contact with mental health professionals. There is no doubt that positive risk taking is necessary in order to move on, to develop and to transcend the role of psychiatric patient. Many survivors of the psychiatric system talk of acts of non-compliance being a necessary turning point in their recovery (Chamberlin 1999). Non-adherence to a care plan that is not fully 'owned' or to a medication regimen that has not been arrived at through informed agreement can be indicative of the spirit of recovery. Non-compliance can be seen as an expression of the individual's per-sonal power, as indicative of their desire to take responsibility for themselves and their lives and to claim a different identity to the one assigned to them by mental health professionals. The key to the ethics of this dilemma is that risk assessment must always be a collaborative process involving all those involved. It should take place within the context of a relationship which is empathic, enabling and respectful. The danger exists of defensive practices emerging to the detriment of the recovery process in services where systems of staff support and supervision are not in place and where the parent organisation does not support the imperative of positive risk taking.

Refusing the call

The call may be refused many times before it is answered positively. People can for a time seem stuck in recurring cycles of acute distress and re-admission or live a clinically managed, symptom-free life but at a low level of functioning. Nothing changes, despite the best efforts of the care team. Such a situation can generate a sense of helplessness, hopelessness and failure among mental health profes-sionals who may project the blame onto the client for the unchanging state of affairs. We need to ask ourselves whether we are part of the problem rather than part of the solution. Are we able to look at the recurrence of distressed, disturbed behaviour as the increasingly urgent promptings of a troubled psyche urging a person to seek a way of being in the world more conducive to wellbeing? Can we see it as an opportunity for helping someone gain more understanding of their distress and for growth and change? Or do we convey the attitude of resignation at the inevitability of relapses and continued vulnerability, a prognosis that can only be improved by the right medication taken reliably? To feel in the grip of something so powerful and pathological from which only equally powerful drugs can set you free is bound to leave people feeling passive victims unable to act in response to the call to embark on a recovery journey. As Gergen (1990) wisely commented, pathologising psychosocial distress is an 'invitation to infirmity'.

Some avoidance of the recovery journey is understandable. There can be pain and discomfort to endure since the journey means taking responsibility for one's life and drawing on resources and strengths one may not be sure one possesses. The traveller must find an energy and will they are not sure is accessible. The goals may seem unclear or unreachable. There can be anxiety about further breakdowns. It can seem hard to care about yourself and your life. It may be safer not to care than risk further failures. It may seem easier to stay in the passive patient role. This may be a role that has been lived for some time and which feels comfortable and familiar; it may give life some frisson, rescue identity from bland anonymity, legitimise an avoidance of life and allow one to indulge in eccentricities; it results in regular contact with caring professionals and a patient community in which one can find warm acceptance. These gains can be hard to give up, but as Coleman (1999) says in reflection on his own recovery process: 'You need to give up being ill so you can start being recovered'. There is also sometimes a seductive element in 'madness' which casts us into a world that can be enthralling as much as disturbing, a world that can appear more enticing than the impoverished life that seems the alternative (Podvoll 2003). Our psychiatric history can be the dominant narrative in our life and can determine our sense of who we are. To discard our ill selves can precipitate an identity crisis that can only be resolved as another self begins to emerge from alternative narratives. Coleman (1999) sees the emergence of self-awareness, self-acceptance, self-esteem and self-confidence as an essential stepping-stone on the road to recovery.

The plain fact is that there is frequently a bias towards inaction and inertia in human behaviour and in order for recovery work to begin we need to find some way of tilting the bias towards action. Passivity reveals itself as doing nothing when faced with the call to action; or acting aimlessly when a life situation calls for a focused effort; or uncritically accepting the solutions suggested by others, even though we have no real commitment to them. Sometimes passivity is rooted in learned helplessness (Seligman 1975). As the result of exposure (often in childhood) to adverse life experiences over which little control or influence can be exerted, someone may acquire an attitude of learned helplessness which becomes a fixed pattern of behaviour. Faced with the challenge of the call, people will habitually behave in helpless ways even when it is perfectly possible for them to initiate some change. Mental health services have been very good at reinforcing learned helplessness and less successful at inculcating learned resourcefulness (Fig. 3.2). Finally, the bias towards action is further compromised by our skill at sabotaging ourselves – what Egan (2002) refers to as disabling self-talk. Often our inner critic will render us speechless and passive in situations that call for a response. This self-imposed impotence gradually undermines self-confidence and social effectiveness and leads to us avoiding life.

The recovery journey can only begin when we have identified and addressed these barriers to change. Inherently people are enormously powerful, resourceful and creative. How could we have survived and prospered as a species were it not so? The task of mental health professionals in helping people to answer the call positively – saying yes to life – is to cultivate self-efficacy. This can be achieved through believing in people; through maintaining a hopeful attitude; through a focus on strengths rather than weaknesses; through helping people to imagine a different future for themselves and to establish achievable goals. At the beginning of every journey, whether inner or outer, there will be anxiety.

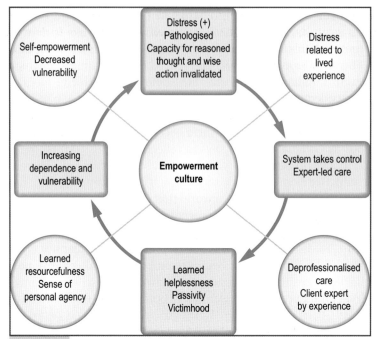

Figure 3.2 Cycle of disempowerment and the counter culture.

Sometimes this anxiety prevents people leaving the safety of a familiar world. A *secure base* provided by relationships – and a relationship with a mental health professional is often of key importance here – enables people to take the first tentative steps in response to the call.

The mentor and the hero's journey

'Mentor' is a term derived from a character in *The Odyssey*. Mentor was Odysseus' loyal friend, entrusted with the guardianship of his family while he was away on his epic journey. In modern mythic stories, such as *Star Wars* and *Lord of the Rings*, we again see the enabling role of the mentor. Mentors may strengthen the will, confidence and fortitude of the traveller and even accompany them for part of the journey. They are the guardians of hopefulness. They entreat the hero to trust himself; to trust that he will find the wisdom and resourcefulness within to come through. Mentors have knowledge of the quest and the journey the person is about to make, often from personal experience. They are able to make a gift of that knowledge and teach the skills a person will need on their journey. Often the hero may have an internalised image of the mentor which helps them during perilous moments in their quest, representing qualities that the hero aspires to. In the context of a recovery journey, this important role may be taken on by family, friends, other service users/survivors, independent advocates, or professional mental health workers.

What are the qualities embodied in a mentor which can help someone set out on and continue their recovery journey? More than anything these are to do with being accessible and available over time; with believing in a person's capacity to grow and change; with developing a relationship which provides what Bowlby (1988) referred to as a 'secure base' from which they can set off in search of a different way of being. Breggin (1997) powerfully describes the nature of this relationship as the 'creation of healing presence'. He argues that the art of being helpful has more to do with being in a certain way with people rather than what we might do:

> To create a healing presence we must fine tune our inner experience to the inner state of the other person, our response then becomes more attuned to the basic needs of the person we are trying to heal and help. Ultimately we find within ourselves the psychological and spiritual resources required to nourish and empower the other human being. (p. 5)

In Breggin's view the ultimate goal of helping deeply disturbed people is the discovery that life can be handled, that out of emotional overwhelming experiences comes growth and the capacity to be a healing presence for ourselves. The strengthening presence of a mentor who is able to relate with a high degree of empathy, acceptance and positive regard can mark a turning point for clients in their recovery journey.

Edward Podvoll, an American psychiatrist and psychotherapist and founder and director of the innovative Windhorse project which provides a 'home based' alternative to orthodox psychiatric treatment, creating recovery environments for people trapped in a world of psychotic experience, has written illuminatingly about recovery relationships (Podvoll 2003). He argues that the 'fragile and tentative drama of recovery' is most likely to come from the 'catalyst of human intimacy'. Central to the recovery environment is the treatment team, a small group of individuals – not necessarily trained mental health professionals – who offer the client 'basic attendance' through regular contact. *Basic attendance* is a therapeutic attitude seen as conducive to recovery. Podvoll describes the interpersonal attributes of basic attendance as *being present; letting in; letting be; bringing home; bringing along; recognising; finding energy; leaning in; discovering friendship; and learning.*

Being present means that when we are with people we have as much of our attention free for them as is possible. Sometimes we may find that our attention is elsewhere, held by our own concerns or sunk in our own distress. In these instances we need to find a way of letting go of those preoccupations on a temporary basis, bringing our attention out so that it is available to the client. Being present is not characterised by an intense focus on the person we are with, but more by a relaxed awareness. Podvoll likens it to a meditative state in which our attention may drift and be caught by some inner experience but that we simply have to acknowledge that drift and bring our attention back to being present in the here and now with the person in our care. It is a quality appreciated by clients and to which they are receptive, even if at the time they are unable to be actively responsive.

Letting in is the skill of being open to the experience of the client's psychological world. We tend to reflexively put up barriers to the emotional distress of others in order to protect ourselves against becoming overwhelmed by the intensity of their experience. Taken to extremes, this can communicate a certain coldness or detachment or reveal itself in an impatient, critical attitude towards the client. But usually such barriers are semi-permeable and we take in the emotional state of the client, whether they are expressing it overtly or not. As many clients find it difficult to communicate the fullness of their inner experience, letting in offers a valuable insight into a client's affective world. Most of us will have experienced ending contact with a client feeling worried and anxious, or angry and aggrieved, or perhaps caught up in a feeling of despondency and hopelessness, or helplessness and powerlessness, and with a sense that this is not our own emotional baggage. It illustrates how important supervision and informal structures that provide an opportunity for reflection on our work actually are. Podvoll argues that letting in is the *birthplace of compassion and deeper empathy.* It allows us to make real contact with the client and to be with them in the psychological place in which they find themselves. Only through reaching people where they are can we help them slip the manacles of the mind and reconnect with the world.

Letting be is a similar interpersonal dynamic to the above, having an inner dimension that reflects in our way of being with clients. If we get too attached to what we think should be happening in the recovery process then we are unlikely to be present with the client with any degree of equanimity. Recovery is never a straightforward process. There are always steps forward and steps backwards. If we invest too much in a positive response to our care, we can burden clients with our expectations. We can also end up feeling frustrated and irritated, blaming the client for their lack of progress or conversely castigating ourselves for being an inadequate, unskilled caregiver. We need to give up our therapeutic egos and maintain a non-judgemental openness to what is.

The interpersonal approach Podvoll refers to as *bringing home* means that we seek to ground people in the reality of everyday life events. Cleaning the toilet, doing your washing, preparing a meal, paying your utility bills – all these make up the fabric of everyday life and ground us in the material world, preventing us from drifting off into a sea of 'madness'. Sharing activities with clients is thus an important pillar of recovery, and enabling them to sufficiently overcome apathy or distraction so as to retain some structure to their life prevents them sliding into chaos.

Bringing along is a development that happens after the initial engagement phase when the relationship has begun to deepen and there is more mutuality. The client may be ready to do more and there is an opportunity to share recreational activities and interests. After years of living an impoverished, isolated life it can be hard for people to re-enter a social world of interests and pleasures and the sanctuary of their shut in world may still seem enticing. It is good to be able to bring people along to things that we ourselves find interesting and enjoyable. There are of course boundary issues here, but I sometimes feel we are too fixated and rigid about boundaries. Of course there must be limits for ethical practice to be maintained, but it has not been my experience that going with clients to football matches, the cinema or art galleries, sometimes outside of contact hours, has compromised my professional relationships.

The nature of therapeutic relationships in which the style of relating can be described as 'person to person' rather than 'worker to patient' brings into focus the issue of friendships in helping relationships (Watkins 2001). Can friendship be discovered in what is essentially a therapeutic encounter? Podvoll argues that 'within the intimacy of basic attendance friendly feelings develop; this is inescapable'. What matters is how that dynamic is perceived and managed. If the issues it raises can be openly acknowledged and worked with so that the recovery process is advanced rather than impeded, all well and good. To deny friendly feelings is to obscure the humanity at the heart of helping relationships beneath a mantle of professionalism.

Finding energy can be a big problem for people sunk in distress who may also be taking large doses of soporific medication. Apathy and inertia can descend on their lives and it can be hard to break out. Yet we know if we reflect on our own lives that to engage in something when we are immersed in a prevailing feeling of lethargy and disinterest can unexpectedly release a flow of energy and stimulate our minds. People can be 'awakened' to life through nature, music, art, food and drink; by the energies of another person; by a sexual frisson; by curiosity; by a desire to recapture a sense of wellbeing; by a desire to bring some order to the chaos of their lives; by an awareness of social expectation and responsibility. Motivation is not something that simply arises from within in response to a pressing unmet need but can be co-created in the drama of interpersonal life.

In recovery relationships with clients we frequently encounter what Podvoll calls 'islands of clarity'. These are moments, sometimes transient, sometimes more sustained, when people seem to escape the clutches of their psychotic world and begin to engage in a shared reality. At these times a person's 'history of sanity' comes into view as the persona of 'madness' leaves the stage, albeit temporarily. At these times people may come face to face with their neglected lives, with the chaos, with the emptiness, with the unfulfilled nature of it; face to face with the self-absorption of their lives and their neglect of a more social, compassionate way of being. This can of course be overwhelmingly dispiriting, but it can also galvanise people into action, enabling them to find the courage and the discipline to cross the threshold and begin the journey of transcending their disorderly mind and transforming their lives. It is vitally important that these *islands of clarity* are recognised by mental health professionals as potential turning points and worked with.

One of the satisfactions of mental health work is when people stop leaning on others and begin to seize responsibility for their lives, what Podvoll calls *leaning in*. The recognition gradually dawns that ultimately no one is responsible for 'fixing their life' but they themselves. To regain autonomy after years during which a person has been entrapped in a dependent role can be difficult. A sense of uncertainty and insecurity invariably surfaces and a retreat into dependency inevitably occurs. But families and professional carers need to be able to stand back sufficiently to allow people to exercise their own judgement, determine their own priorities and meet their own needs, so that they begin to recognise and trust their own inner strength and resourcefulness.

One young man I have come to know has a long history of a disabling thought disorder and has struggled to maintain an autonomous life and adequate self-care. What with the intrusive care by his mother and the intervening care of mental health professionals, he has lost sovereignty over his life and, even when islands of clarity appear in his psychotic confusion, he finds it hard to live well. One of his preoccupations is a misconception of himself as physically small and weak. His thoughts are often about building himself up; becoming bigger and stronger. It is not much of an imaginative leap to see this obsession as a metaphor for his threatened masculinity and his diminished autonomy and personal power. The challenge for us in working with this young man is to make better use of the opportunities provided by the islands of clarity, which seem so often to provoke a sense of the 'impossibility' of resurrecting his life with the result that he succumbs once more to the 'seduction of madness'. We are working collaboratively with him to *bring home* the value of self-care, the maintenance of his flat and the creation of a home. We are *bringing him along* to a life of interest and pleasure within the wider community so that reconnecting to a life of sanity will ground him more securely in the rational, material world.

As mental health workers we are privileged. We can learn much from our care of clients on their recovery journeys. So much of what we witness in the struggles of people to regain their wellbeing and recover their lives will have meaning for us personally in our own quest for growth and a life well lived. We can learn to apply the attitudes of basic attendance to ourselves: attending to ourselves; letting in and acknowledging our innermost feelings and needs; grounding ourselves mindfully in the routine of daily living; weaving into the fabric of our lives sources of pleasure and satisfaction; taking responsibility for our lives; finding within ourselves the spirit to act with loving kindness towards others; locating within the courage and the discipline to realise more of our potential.

These ways of relating can be adopted and developed by anyone involved in the recovery care of the client, whether a mental health professional or not. They are interpersonal qualities rather than intervention skills. They are in my view the cornerstone of recovery work and I am indebted to Edward Podvoll for providing the vision of how therapeutic relationships with people adrift in psychological turmoil can be.

We will say more in Chapter 8 about 'Recovery relationships'.

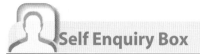

Self Enquiry Box

Think for a moment about who you would want around you should you begin experiencing an excitation of the mind; if you were being drawn into a delusional world; if your thoughts became disconnected and confused; if you began to experience troubling voices; if your volitional energy became dissipated and you drifted into apathy and inertia.

- Who would you like to have in your recovery team?
- You may be able to think of specific people. Think about the qualities and attributes they possess which you think would help you recover.

You might find it helpful to consider which of those qualities you identify as desirable in your personal recovery team you are able to bring to your own recovery work with clients and which you need to develop. Now consider

- What would be your ideal recovery environment? What specific features would be most important to you?
- How many of the features of your ideal recovery environment are available in the environments of clients you work with?

Crossing the threshold

Quest: to set out in pursuit of goals with determination, courage and hopefulness

The threshold is the stage when people begin seriously to contemplate the recovery journey, to imagine a different future for themselves. 'When I'm feeling better about my life and myself what will be present in my life that's not present now?' 'When I am coping better with my problems of living what will I be doing that I'm not doing now?' These are crucial questions. Taking people to the threshold of change offers a vista of a life which is different, where possibilities and opportunities can be explored. It can be a turning point, an experience that releases people from a prevailing sense of hopelessness about themselves and their lives. It is a satisfying moment in helping relationships when someone seizes the moment and makes a commitment to the pursuit of life-changing goals.

For some people, turning points seem to come at moments when things 'can't get much worse'. It is there, in that desolation, that the will to be well returns; as in addiction, where it is not until people can no longer avoid facing the wreckage of their lives and their powerlessness to change things alone that the process of recovery can begin. For others the catalyst may be a loving relationship within which they find a reason to begin the task of transcending their 'sick role'. Finding meaning and purpose in life through religion, through educational and employment opportunities, or through creative endeavour can invoke the spirit of change. Some accomplishment or success can also be the stimulus that leads to further incremental steps towards more engagement in life and recovery.

Sometimes it is a decision to stop taking recreational drugs or using alcohol that signals a desire to, as one service user put it, 'sort my head out and my life too'. For a significant number of people the continued use of cannabis, crack cocaine or amphetamines seriously undermines their attempts to cross the threshold. A turning point may also be heralded by a collaborative decision to change, or beginning to use a medication that helps in the management of symptoms sufficiently for a person to start rebuilding the fabric of their life. Finally, sometimes that elusive turning point is only reached when people step away from mental health services so that a new embryonic identity can begin to emerge and emotional emancipation can be experienced. Turning points can take several years to reach but research into recovery from serious and enduring mental health problems suggests that no one is beyond hope. For the complexity of reasons we have discussed in this chapter it may be five, 10, perhaps 15 years, perhaps longer, before the psychological turmoil clears sufficiently to reveal a person's potential qualities and strengths which have remained, waiting to be uncovered.

Even at the point of crossing the threshold it can be difficult to take the next step, to respond to the call to step away from a life as a 'career patient' and face the challenges of life with all its struggles and responsibilities as well as its joys. Many people continue to feel a deep sense of disempowerment, and are still lacking the confidence and self-esteem to strike out in the direction of their dreams. Years of problem-orientated care can result in them being overly conscious of their vulnerabilities and disabilities, as a consequence of which they will have lost touch with their resourcefulness, skills and strengths. The life story within which a person defines her/himself may have become problem laden, where the central character is seen as a failure, as inadequate and helpless, or as a victim – a self-definition from which it is difficult to start a recovery journey. White (1995) emphasises the importance of rescuing normalcy from pathology, suggesting there is always a richer narrative to be found in the obscured story lines of a person's life which can be the basis for a redefinition of self, a self with qualities and strengths that the individual has lost sight of in their emotionally overwhelmed state. Being on the threshold of change can therefore be very anxiety provoking, leading to self-questioning – 'Will I be able to cope, will I fail, will I be able to find acceptance, friendship, love? What will I do in the wider community beyond the cloistered psychiatric system? Will the demands of living precipitate another breakdown?' As we have seen, a mentor can be a key figure in determining whether someone crosses the threshold and sets out with determination, courage and hopefulness – a recovery relationship in which someone believes in that person's potential and worth, who cares and extends to them what Deegan (1988) has called 'a loving invitation to be something more'.

The way to recovery

Quest: overcoming doubts, fears, obstacles and setbacks to reach our goal

The journey of recovery, as we have seen, is not about finding a cure for psychological distress and dysfunction. Such a brave new world, were it remotely possible, would rob us of our humanity – to be human is to experience both suffering and joy. What we need to be concerned with is a way of being in the world that is less problematic and more fulfilling; a way of finding within ourselves the spirit and the qualities that allow us to transcend diagnostic labels and archaic distress. It involves a process of accepting what has happened to us and discovering meaning in it. It is about forgiving ourselves and others and liberating the wondrous parts of ourselves that have been obscured by our distress and embracing a life not circumscribed by negativity and misfortune.

In reviewing personal testimonies in the recovery literature Davidson (2003) identifies commonalities in the journeys of individuals that seem to capture the essence of recovery. These include:

- redefining self
- accepting vulnerabilities
- overcoming stigma
- regaining hope
- resuming control and responsibility for one's life
- exercising citizenship
- managing continuing or recurrent manifestations of distress
- experiencing the love and support of others
- involvement in meaningful activities and expanded social roles.

There are many pathways to the realisation of these conditions for a less troubled, more enriched life and a sustainable sense of wellbeing. In this section and in subsequent chapters we will look in some detail at the therapies, strategies and supports which people use on the way to recovery. A study by the Mental Health Foundation (2000) has thrown some light on what people find *most helpful* on their way to recovery (Box 3.4). What is clear is that the strategies for managing distress, rebuilding identities and reclaiming life have the stamp of individuality on them.

Box 3.4

Service users' views of factors most helpful in recovery

- Relationships with friends, family, other service users, mental health professionals
- Safe havens; accepting communities; shared experience/identities with others; accessible/available support
- Finding meaning and purpose through: family; work; meaningful activity; helping others; creative expression; religion or spiritual practice
- Use of medication; psychotherapy; complementary therapies; arts therapies; exercise; communion with nature
- Being in control of one's vulnerability to distress; being in control of one's life; having enough money; having secure accommodation; finding pleasure in life

Adapted from Mental Health Foundation study (2000)

There has long been a misconception among mental health professionals that people are passive victims of their distress. Nothing could be further from the truth. People adopt their own strategies to try and regain emotional equilibrium and peace of mind. Some of these are constructive and helpful in providing relief and promoting recovery. Others may not work or may just give some temporary relief, or may be maladaptive or damaging. Working with people to identify what works for them and how to maximise those strategies is a key intervention in enabling clients to feel more in control and empowered in managing their distress experience.

The predominant theme running through people's recovery testimonies is the value of relationships with friends and family, other service users and mental health professionals. Many people have found programmes led by service users and survivors and voluntary sector projects such as those run by local Mind associations an important source of help and empowerment in their journey (Ahern & Fisher 2001). Within this social context people are often able to find the acceptance, sense of belonging, companionship and friendship that are missing in the wider community (Mental Health Foundation 2000). Ingrained in voluntary sector services, though sadly often absent from the statutory provision, is a belief in the potential of people to achieve a fulfilled life whatever their history – as Nietzsche so poetically put it, 'Only out of chaos may there be born a dancing star'.

The complementary or alternative way

There has been a significant shift in Western culture towards a more holistic way of thinking about wellness. We recognise the need for balance and harmony in the physical, psychological, spiritual, social and ecological dimensions of our lives. There is disenchantment with conventional medicine which often fails to deliver desired outcomes in persistent and recurrent health problems and a distrust of pharmacological interventions. As a result, holistic therapies have become significant in the recovery journey of many people. A study by the Mental Health Foundation (1997, 2000) of a heterogeneous group of service users found that over 85% had experienced complementary therapies and found them helpful or helpful at times, a satisfaction level far higher than that for prescribed medication. Of those using complementary therapies, 20% found a combination of therapies (for example a talking therapy and an exercise/postural therapy such as yoga) to be the most helpful factor in the recovery of wellbeing. People clearly appreciated the holistic nature of therapies – the experience of being treated *as a whole person* and in a *person-centred way*. Many people like the empowering sense of being active in their own healing process, of having responsibility for the reclamation of their mental health. For most people, holistic therapies offered a way of managing anxiety and depression through the *relaxation, calm, balance and harmony* achieved in and beyond a treatment session. The therapies contributed to a sense of being grounded and centred rather than being *all over the place,* resulting in an improvement in cognitive functioning, while the compassionate way of being and relating of holistic practitioners is valued by clients, with the calm, unhurried ambience of the therapeutic encounter contributing to the overall benefit. Interventions that release our inherent capacity for self-healing are widely regarded as a more natural and acceptable way to restore wellbeing than pharmacologically orientated psychiatry. Even so, the majority of people see holistic therapies as being complementary to orthodox psychiatric treatment rather than an alternative, although for some, including a contributor to this book, they have been the mainstay of recovery.

The Mental Health Foundation study revealed the wide range of therapies used. These include: acupuncture, reflexology, aromatherapy massage, reiki, yoga, tai chi, Alexander technique, homeopathy, herbalism and healing. The choice of therapy was mostly determined by personal preference and availability rather than known efficacy. The appropriateness of a therapy for an individual is important. For some people (for example those who have had negative experiences of touch, associating it with violence or sexual assault), the intimacy of physical therapies such as massage can be threatening. Conversely gentle touch can be experienced as emotionally sustaining and self-affirming to people who have little intimate contact in their lives and whose tactile needs are not being met. One participant in the study, commenting on a massage session, said 'I found it really comforting and warm and almost fell asleep having been all tense and frightened. It was like – oh I feel great!' Many people hold emotional tension in their musculature – it is literally the embodiment of our mental defences. Releasing this tension can bring into awareness the distress previously suppressed. As one respondent in the study reported: 'It released so much in my body, from what had happened in the past and brought everything up to the surface, in a way talking never had.' An emotional discharge from old wounds can of course be healing, but the therapist needs to have the necessary skills to contain strong feelings and help the client process the reaction. This is why many people find it hard to allow themselves to relax in relaxation classes. To do so would be to risk being defenceless against feelings and fears that threaten to engulf them. It is preferable for some people to achieve anxiety reduction and relaxation through more active strategies such as tai chi, yoga and the practice of meditation. This is reflected in the experience of two of the study's respondents:

Meditation I've found useful, it helps you be aware of the moment rather than worrying about what's going to happen next week ...

Tai chi was so relaxing it somehow cleared your mind. You had to concentrate on learning the movements and that took your mind off your problems – or maybe it was the movements themselves – whatever it was it had a positive effect.

There are two main problems involved in integrating holistic therapies more fully into recovery work. The first is the lack of a good research base providing evidence of their efficacy, which in the arena of evidence-based National Health Service (NHS) psychiatry has resulted in complementary medicine being somewhat peripheral to treatment/care plans. There have been some well conducted randomised controlled trials of acupuncture in the treatment of major depression which suggest significant benefits in terms of relief of symptoms and recovery time compared with antidepressant treatment (Allen et al 1998; Roschke et al 2000). Research into the herbal treatment of mild to moderate depression with St John's wort has shown it to be as effective as antidepressants (Fava et al 2005; Demling et al 2004). In a review of the evidence for homeopathy Reilly (2005) makes a strong claim for the value of homeopathic medicine in recovery from depression and states of anxiety.

More imaginatively designed research studies which meet the accepted criteria for validity and reliability are needed to back up the extensive single personal reflection on recovery reports and the experiential evidence from outcome surveys, both of which make a persuasive case for the value of a wide range of holistic therapies.

The second major problem is that of cost. Except where holistic therapy is available as part of the NHS service provision or available at low cost through non-statutory organisations such as Mind, the cost puts complementary therapy beyond the reach of most clients. Yet it seems to me that the potential benefits in terms of reduced use of medication, improved recovery time, sustained well-being and positive life change more than justify contracting in these services, simply from the point of view of cost-effectiveness, quite apart from consumer satisfaction.

The way of nature

Communion with nature enlivens the spirit, diminishes the preoccupations of the ego and grounds us in the natural world, reminding us that we are all the progeny of Gaia. Following the death of my son, in the deepest phase of my grief, I found in the natural world the promise of healing and recovery. It seemed to affect me at two levels. Firstly it induced me to look up and out, taking my attention out of the distress that was consuming me. On my solitary walks along the shore line close to where I live, it felt as if my wounded psyche was being bathed in the waters of the estuary and my aching heart wrapped in the green folds of the river valley. But it was not always so! At times my sadness was so deadening that I felt disconnected from nature. At these times I believe the effect was subliminal: rather than nature drawing me out, it was entering me, resonating with that which is indomitable in both humankind and the natural world. The naturalist Richard Mabey describes a similar process in his recovery from severe depression: 'What healed me I think was a sense of being not taken out of myself but back in, of nature entering me, firing up the wild bits of my imagination' (Mabey 2005).

In a small study of the effect of restorative environments on a service user group, Priest (2006) found evidence that walking in the countryside can have the effect of making the walker feel *soothed, relieved and restored*. One member of the group involved in the study who had experienced overwhelming distress and threatening voices following a gang rape commented that 'you don't need to put up barriers against nature because its there to love you as much as you love her'. She describes how, while walking, she found herself 'dissolving into the landscape' and that the experience of merging with something infinitely bigger than herself helped disperse her pain.

Over the past decade ecopsychology has begun to have some impact on the thinking of psychologists and psychiatrists. The conception of the biophilic nature of man – that is the evolutionary based affiliation of humankind with the natural world, a natural world from which we have become estranged – is gaining some support. Although clinicians continue to seek the cause of psychological disturbances within the individual, or less commonly within the family system and less commonly still within society, there is the seed of recognition that we have to widen the sphere of enquiry to include the natural world, of which we are a part, if we are going to comprehend the levels of distress that are currently being seen.

Because of our estrangement from the natural world, our arrogant, exploitative, destructive attitude towards it continues unrestrained and is reflected in the disease we experience as a species (Roszak et al 1995). Is it taking this line of reasoning a step too far to suggest that as a species we are the consciousness of nature and that in damaging the world we are damaging ourselves? The distress that we feel about what we have done and are doing to the biosphere – the rape of Gaia – manifests itself in the increasing incidence of mental health problems. Though this is subject to denial (how could we face the enormity of the fear and the grief?), we must make it conscious, work through our sense of despair and powerlessness and reconnect with the benevolence and beauty of nature of which we are a part. It is only through the reunion and communion with the natural world that we will heal the world and ourselves.

The psychotherapeutic way

A myriad of models of psychotherapeutic practice are available in the UK, though not necessarily accessible to people with severe mental health problems.

This is partly because of the pharmacological grip on the thinking of mental health professionals. Neuroleptic medication is always seen as the first line of treatment – and sometimes the second and third lines too. Added to this is the persistent but erroneous belief that, with the exception of cognitive behavioural therapy, psychotherapeutic interventions are of limited therapeutic value in severe and persistent mental health problems.

The debate continues about the value of specificity in psychotherapeutic interventions. In other words, are some strategies more effective than others in relieving distress symptoms? In a significant overview of psychotherapies Hubble et al (1999) showed that the actual techniques of psychotherapy accounted for less than 15% of the change in clients; 15% was attributed to the placebo effect; the relationship with the therapist was seen as responsible for 30% of the change; and 40% of the outcome depended on clients themselves. Hubble and his colleagues concluded that 'the clients' own generative self-healing capacities allow them to take what therapies have to offer and use them to self-heal'. Despite the widespread belief in the 'magical power of therapy' to heal one's psyche and mend one's life, it seems clear that the only magic – and it is powerful magic – is the client's propensity for self-healing which is mobilised in the therapy session.

It is clear from surveys of resources used by mental health service users that 'talking therapies' are highly valued, and experienced by most people as beneficial (Mental Health Foundation 1997, 2000). What people find beneficial about psychotherapeutic interventions ranges from the tangible to the less tangible (though the latter should not be underestimated):

> It's helped me manage my voices; make sense of my experience; reduce my medication; feel more in control of my life and recovery; taught me to cope with stressful situations; improved my confidence and self-esteem; it helped me accept myself; I was able to release emotional tension; I was able to talk about the things I needed to talk about; I was treated as a whole person; it was like having someone alongside supporting you; being listened to, believed and understood was reassuring; it helped me heal the wounds I suffered in the past; helped me understand the roots of my mental illness in the emotional damage I had experienced; helped me look at things – my hypersensitivities, in another way; helped me understand and learn strategies for coping with my depression.

It is possible to conclude from this snapshot of outcomes that people faced with a vulnerability to recurrent episodes of psychological turmoil and social disruption could, as the Hubble et al study suggests, potentially find any psychotherapeutic intervention helpful, whatever its theoretical orientation. All schools of psychotherapy would claim these process experiences to be integral to their model and the stated outcomes achievable. The facilitating factor common to all therapy is the creation of a calm, safe, therapeutic space where a person can think and talk about their experiences in the presence of a therapist who is perceived as being authentic, non-judgemental and empathic and who is committed to being a compassionate ally in the process of change and recovery. But beyond these commonalities there are differences in the theory and practice of facilitating change and it is important that people are able to access good information about the various psychotherapeutic modalities so that choice can be exercised.

In Chapter 8, 'Recovery relationships', I will argue that person-centred psychotherapeutic helping contributes significantly to positive outcomes in states of psychological overwhelm. In this section I will briefly discuss the development of cognitive behavioural therapy (CBT) as a way forward in the recovery journey.

It has been argued by Chadwick et al (1996) that CBT normalises psychotic phenomena by positing continuity between what might be described as a psychotic experience, such as a delusional belief, and the unusual beliefs held by many people who are not considered psychotic. I would not want to play down the extreme and divergent nature of some beliefs, for example that a television news item carries a coded message for you, or that you are a member of the Special Air Services counter-insurgency unit, but simply to underline that such unusual and disturbing beliefs are often understandable in the context of the person's life and developmental history. Chadwick et al make a case for redefining psychotic symptoms – unshackling them from a symptom model and instead seeking to understand such unusual manifestations of human experience in relation to the psychology of the person.

Similarly Romme & Escher, in their groundbreaking studies of voice hearing, demonstrated conclusively that hearing voices is a widely distributed phenomenon, not exclusively associated with psychiatric morbidity (Romme & Escher 1989, 1993). What is significant is the association between voice hearing and a previous experience of trauma or deprivation, exacerbated by current stressors, reported by 70% of voice hearers, both diagnosed and undiagnosed (Pennings & Romme 1998). A characterising difference between voice hearers who have a psychiatric diagnosis and those who are non-patients is that the former group are more likely to experience voices in a predominantly negative way and are more fearful of them. Their daily lives are often significantly disrupted by voices and they feel powerless to influence them. This contrasts strikingly with the 'non-patient' voice hearers who have a predominantly positive experience of voices, experience less distress and feel more in control. These findings have had a significant influence on approaches to understanding and working with voices and led to the setting up of the British Voice Hearers Network in 1990. The network aims to de-stigmatise voice hearing through education and the promotion of alternative explanations, to develop strategies for coping with voices and empower people to live with the experience in positive ways. In pursuit of these aims, voice hearers' self-help groups have mushroomed around the country.

Although CBT as a strategy for coping with voices and delusions has a relatively short history, the approach has its roots in the seminal work of Aaron Beck dating from four decades ago, an approach that has been widely used with success in the treatment of depression and anxiety related problems. Accumulating evidence suggests that cognitive therapy for psychotic experiences is as effective as cognitive interventions for emotional disorders and that those improvements are maintained (Rector & Beck 2002). Delusional thinking reflects a tendency towards an egocentric bias in the way a person perceives the world. Events, particularly those that are emotionally salient, are ascribed an unjustified personal relevance. Uncorrected, the distorting lens through which events are viewed leads to the formation of rigid beliefs of an unusual nature which may be distressing and have a profound effect on an individual's behaviour. The therapeutic process involves an exploration of an individual's personal history out of which the delusional ideas have emerged, an identification of the triggers for delusional thinking and the emotional and behavioural reactions to those intrusive, troubling thoughts. The essence of the CBT approach is to sow seeds of doubt about the validity of dysfunctional beliefs, by supportively challenging people to consider alternative explanations and to question their previously held interpretations, inferences and predictions.

As in the case of delusions, the CBT approach to managing voices starts with a collaborative enquiry into the origin of a person's hallucinatory experience – the experience of raw vulnerability from which the voices sprang. The exploratory discussion encompasses the content of the voices, beliefs about them, the circumstances which lead to an increase in voice hearing and how the person reacts to the hallucinatory experience. The latter line of enquiry may identify ways in which the individual is currently managing their voices so that the distress and interference they cause is reduced. The current focus of CBT in the management of voices has been to weaken the omnipotence and omniscience of voices by helping people develop strategies to exert more control over them by eliciting alternative perspectives on the voice content and the beliefs about the voices. A number of strategies have been successfully used by voice hearers:

Dialogue within a recovery relationship

There is no doubt that an accepting relationship in which there is genuine empathic interest can provide a helpful basis for a dialogue in which voice hearing experiences can be collaboratively explored and worked with. This is in contrast to the received wisdom of the past which held that, apart from the purpose of assessment and diagnosis, interactions with clients should deflect attention away from psychotic phenomena, thus helping them become more grounded in everyday reality. As a result, some people have spent years tormented by voices, feeling powerless and isolated:

> It was only after 15 years of psychiatric interventions I was able to find someone willing to listen. This proved a turning point for me and from this I was able to break out of being a victim and start owning my experience ... she helped me realise that the voices were part of me and had purpose and validity. Over a six month period I was able to develop a basic strategy for coping. (Cited in Romme & Escher 1993)

Keeping a diary

It is not always possible to confide in others about voices. Janet, one of the contributors to this book, was forbidden by her voices to talk to anyone about them and was not able to share her experience for 10 years. Diary keeping can be a way of discharging feelings, of distracting oneself from intrusive voices, of understanding voice hearing experiences – the nature of the voices, the triggers, the content and meaning; and the degree of influence and control over voices or the powerlessness one feels. As one voice hearer commented, 'Recently I have come to understand what my voices mean and my diary has played a big part in this respect'. Sometimes too a diary can provide a useful basis for dialogue between a person and their mental health worker.

Talking back to voices

Most of us are conscious of an inner dialogue taking place in our minds at various times. It is as if there is in our psychological make-up an assembly of selves or sub-personalities, some of which become energised and express themselves and others which we disown and keep hidden. Voices can be conceptualised in this way as an energised and vocal sub-personality which has broken through our defences – perhaps at a time of stress – and into consciousness. Because it is disowned, it is experienced as other than ourselves. Accepting and dialoguing with voices can therefore lead to increased awareness of a facet of ourselves that needs acknowledging and integrating. As a person begins to feel less powerless in the face of omnipotent voices, it may be possible to tell the voices to stop or to negotiate periods of time for engaging with them. One voice hearer said, 'I've learned to give "the critic" full rein then after a bit it loses its energy and I can tell it to fuck off – which it does'.

Anxiety management

The experience of many voice hearers is that voices are more intrusive at times of stress and anxiety. Anxiety management strategies may therefore be valuable in coping with voices. Taking a yoga or tai chi class or learning mindfulness meditation skills can be helpful. Sometimes voices will become louder and interfere in classes or practice. If this is the case, more active or distracting pursuits such as listening to music may achieve some relief and relaxation. Much of the anxiety that people experience in relation to voices is associated with the power and negativity of voices, their bewildering nature and the degree to which they intrude and interfere with life. For most people, anxiety is reduced when they feel less alone with their voices, have more understanding of the origin and meaning of the voices and feel more in control. One client who frequently hears a voice telling him to commit acts of violence needs to have his own power and control reinforced and strengthened by support workers to allay his anxieties. For some people, dealing with the anxiety caused by the content of voices is the main issue. In this situation CBT strategies which dispute the content of the voices and clarify internal beliefs which serve as self-validation and as a countermand to the voices can be helpful. Sometimes anxiety can be more situational. The intrusion and interference of voices at work, or during conversations with friends and family can cause anxiety and the help needed might be to have more control over voices in those particular circumstances.

A voice hearer known to me experienced episodes of high level anxiety and panic associated with the voice of a computer that he believed had been implanted in his brain. The voice threatened to stop his heart, damage his brain or make him impotent, threats which seemed so menacingly real that he often referred himself for medical help. Bearing in mind that voices can sometimes be thought of as metaphors for some denied aspect of ourselves and our experience, the emotionless nature of the computer voice seems significant in the case of this person. His voices began after the sudden death of his mother, a loss which he had never fully grieved. The image of her death 'implanted' in his memory had resulted in him becoming mindless, heartbroken and less vital, signs which were apparent in his distracted, shut down state.

Voice hearers' groups

Self-help groups, mostly affiliated to the Voice Hearers' Network, have mushroomed around Britain, a development that has been seen as a direct reaction to orthodox psychiatry's pathogenic approach to voice hearing. In the voice hearers' group, the sufferer gets and gives the kind of help that is often missing from mental health care. The group offers a forum where people can talk about their voices, find support and companionship with others who have similar experiences, learn how to live with the experience of voices and explore the meaning of voices – all of which can contribute to the dissipation of the fear and isolation that voice hearing causes.

Although the evidence for the effectiveness of CBT in reducing residual psychotic experiences is significant, it is not invariably successful and even when it is successful does not always lead to an improvement in social functioning and quality of life (Garety et al 2000). In a development of the CBT model Tarrier & Calam (2002) place greater emphasis on the interpersonal and social consequence of voice hearing and delusional thinking. Their approach, functional cognitive behavioural therapy (FCBT), is less concerned with challenging cognitive distortion and more concerned with how unusual beliefs, voices and negative symptoms interfere with the person's ability to engage in life. The therapeutic process involves identifying functional goals and subsequently exploring the way in which psychotic phenomena and barriers to social integration, such as stigma and low self-esteem, make realising those aspirations difficult. Such goals might be making friends or personal relationships, obtaining part-time work or volunteering, attending a leisure learning course, going to public places such as a café, library, cinema or shop, or becoming a member of a gym. The strategies to reduce the interference of symptoms may be similar to more traditional CBT interventions but their goal is not symptom alleviation but improved social functioning and social integration, a shift in focus that can be motivational.

The pursuit of pleasurable activities enhances a sense of wellbeing but it can be difficult for some people after years of impoverished living to reconnect with sources of pleasure or to adopt a hopeful attitude towards its attainment. Fava et al (1998) suggest that people might need encouragement to reflect on periods of wellbeing and to identify experiences and activities that represent sources of positive feeling. Sometimes the use of a pleasure list can be useful if people find it difficult to generate life-enhancing goals.

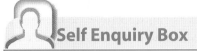

Self Enquiry Box

- Think of 20 things that give you pleasure and promote a sense of wellbeing. List them.
- Now ask yourself how often you allow yourself these pleasures: frequently? occasionally? rarely?
- Consider whether they are pleasures that can be experienced alone, require the presence of others or are a mixture of both.
- Reflect on the personal resources you utilise in order to incorporate these sources of wellbeing into your lifestyle, for example energy, self-esteem and confidence, concentration, sociability and social skills, personal finances, personal transport.
- Finally, identify the barriers that prevent you accessing potential sources of wellbeing.

You might find it useful to complete this exercise yourself before using it as a basis for client work.

The way of mindfulness

Mindfulness is a practice that has its deepest origins in Buddhist philosophy and practice and is prominent in the contemporary teachings of the Vietnamese monk Thich Nhat Hanh, which have a growing following in the West (Thich Nhat Hanh 1991). It should not, however, be thought of as a spiritual practice that is exclusively Buddhist. Indeed, similar practices can be found in the Christian contemplative tradition. In recent times the practice of mindfulness has emerged in the secular world of psychology and has received some attention as a practice for releasing the mind from bondage to troubling thoughts, feelings and perceptual experiences (Hirst 2003). There is some evidence that a mindfulness-based cognitive therapy approach is effective in reducing the incidence of relapse in individuals vulnerable to disabling mental health problems (Segal et al 2002). Mindfulness is the practice of unattached awareness in which the flow of phenomena through consciousness is witnessed in an accepting and dispassionate way. It involves letting go of mental events, not investing them with significance beyond their ephemeral nature. Attachment to, and signification of, the phenomena arising in consciousness is, according to Buddhist teaching, a major cause of unhappiness and suffering. It is not difficult to see how through the attribution of negative meaning a transient thought or feeling can become a fixed object of our consciousness and can disturb our equilibrium. Yet the power of that mental event to disturb us only exists because of the way we embellish it. The practice of mindfulness as a life skill allows us to be more selective about what we pay attention to, allows us to let go of the painful ruminations that can haunt our waking life and frees our mind for living. Through practice, a more detached non-judgemental awareness of the habitual patterns of thinking and feeling to which we react in dysfunctional ways emerges. A more detached stance enables people to calmly and purposefully respond to these harbingers of distress (O'Haver Day & Horton Deutsch 2004).

59

Mindfulness can be taught to individuals or groups and can be integrated into recovery work with people using mental health services. A psycho-educational programme to teach mindfulness would typically involve an exploration of the philosophy and relevance of the practice to mental health, the nature of the practice itself and the barriers to regular practice that individuals might experience. The strategy of becoming a compassionate observer of the self is explored revealing the patterns of thinking and feeling which trigger dysfunctional mood states and behavioural reactions, as well as an awareness of the strengthening joy-filled thoughts that traverse consciousness in day-to-day life. Being more in the here and now rather than the there and then is encouraged through mindful activity and simple meditation such as following the breath (Box 3.5). As a person's capacity for meditative practice increases, a more phlegmatic attitude develops to the mental events that previously precipitated distress symptoms and these can be seen as transient experiences. Practitioners seeking to teach mindfulness would need to deepen their own mindfulness practice through meditation, self-reflection and self-knowledge and undertake training through workshops or certificated teacher training programmes.

Box 3.5

Mindfulness exercise

Write the phrases down and place the paper in front of you. Settle yourself in a quiet space where you will not be disturbed. Start to key into your breathing rhythm, letting it gradually slow down. Then use the following words for the focus of the meditation:

Breathing in, I know I am breathing in.
Breathing out, I know I am breathing out.

Breathing in, my breath grows deep.
Breathing out, my breath goes slowly.

Breathing in, I feel calm.
Breathing out, I feel ease.

Breathing in, I know I am breathing in.
Breathing out, I know I am breathing out.

Adapted from Thich Nhat Hanh (1993)

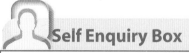

Self Enquiry Box

You will find it useful to practise mindfulness exercises yourself before introducing them to clients. Regular practice will allow you to experience the effect of freeing yourself from the tyranny of negative thoughts and feelings; freeing more of the mind for here and now living. Mindfulness can be practised in everyday situations by first paying attention to the breath to free attention from the preoccupations of the psyche and then allowing the mind to focus on a current activity, such as walking in the garden or washing the dishes, which is carried out in an unhurried, contemplative way, bringing attention back to the focus if distracted by invasive thoughts.

Early intervention and the way to recovery

Early intervention in first episode psychosis has emerged in recent years as of paramount importance in the recovery process. It is not uncommon for people to experience emotional and behavioural difficulties which are the precursors of a more serious breakdown for up to five years before those difficulties develop into the turmoil of psychosis (Johannessen 2004). Even then, the severity and nature of a young person's distress – we are principally talking about a 16–25 age group – can sometimes go unrecognised for a further 1–2 years before an appropriate psychiatric intervention is offered. It is important that a compassionate, recovery-orientated intervention is available and accessible in the prodromal phase or early in the psychotic phase of a person's breakdown because of what Birchwood et al (1998) have referred to as a 'critical window' for maximising the potential for full recovery. The longer psychosis remains untreated, the more entrenched and skewed an individual's self-view and world view become and the more dysfunctional their behaviour. Effective intervention at an early stage can reduce the risk of psychosis occurring (Falloon 1992; McGowry et al 2002) and where a transition to a psychotic episode has already taken place, can reduce the likelihood of further relapses (Power et al 1998). It is not only an improvement in prognosis that makes early detection and intervention an imperative but also because there is a resultant decrease in the risk of suicide, the majority of which take place in the first six years following the onset of psychosis (Mortensen & Juel 1993), and other damaging behaviours such as substance abuse.

What is involved in a compassionate, recovery-orientated intervention in first episode psychosis? While a 'best practice' regimen has yet to emerge from current research, some strong pointers to what is effective have come from the first wave of early intervention programmes. Most advocate an approach which combines an intensive case management model with low-dose antipsychotic medication (Falloon et al 1998). The cornerstone of the approach is the development of a therapeutic relationship between the case manager and the client, a process which takes place within the client's familiar social world. Through this relationship an enormous amount of psychosocial support can be provided. Work on 'triggers', 'relapse signatures' and 'coping strategies' can take place and access to other interventions and services which the client may need to recover and pursue their personal goals can be facilitated. Interventions and services that have been shown to have an influence on recovery and relapse prevention are psychotherapeutic interventions (Gleeson et al 2003), psychoeducational family work (Mullen et al 2002), and access to vocational training or educational opportunities. Engagement with services needs to be sustained over at least two years (Birchwood et al 1998).

A study by O'Toole et al (2004) looked at service users' perspectives on the treatment they received from an early intervention team in the London borough of Southwark. What emerged strongly was the importance of the person-centred relationship that developed between mental health workers and clients in the recovery process. Clients valued the availability of their case managers, felt respected, cared for, listened to and understood. They were involved in treatment decisions, actively supported in structuring their day, and helped in getting their lives 'back on track'. Also seen as important was the mediation work with families.

The strong working alliance with case managers and other members of the team is undoubtedly experienced as a formative relationship during a period in individuals' lives when they feel lost, overwhelmed, confused and frightened. Through these relationships people are able to come to some understanding of their psychological crises, are able to find themselves and reconnect in positive ways with the social fabric of their lives. Johannessen (2004), commenting on developments in early intervention services, underlines the importance of the therapeutic relationship in the following observation:

> We meet people who suffer the deepest possible anxiety, the deepest despair and depression that any human can experience. And we, being therapists, find that in this place before the psychosis and psychotic way of reasoning has tightened its grip, it is easier to talk, easier to relate and easier to re-establish a normal psychological pattern. We see that the social consequences are less devastating, the suffering person has better insight, and the families and social network are better preserved. (p. 331)

The psychopharmacological way

Psychotropic medication in the form of antipsychotic, antidepressant and anxiolytic drugs has been the first line of treatment for severe and persistent mental health problems for the past 50 years. The frequency with which these drugs are prescribed is increasing at an alarming rate. In 1987 there were 2.3 million prescriptions of antipsychotic drugs in Britain. By 2001 there were 5.7 million (Ross & Read 2004). A debate rumbles on and periodically erupts into the public domain about the efficacy and ethics of pharmacological treatment – and there are significant questions to be answered. Are psychotropic drugs essentially benign chemical agents that release people from the bonds of a disturbed state of mind so that they can pursue their lives unfettered or are they hazardous compounds that suppress vitality along with disturbance? Is the powerful pharmaceutical industry unethically exploiting human distress on the basis of questionable research data for commercial success? Has the idea of a 'happiness pill' got such a hold on the thinking of mental health professionals and the general public that we have become too reliant on psychoactive drugs to provide an answer to the problems of living?

As psychiatrists Joanna Moncrief and Phil Thomas openly acknowledge:

> The financial muscle of the pharmaceutical industry has helped tip the scales in favour of a predominantly biological view of psychiatric disorder. This has submerged alternative therapeutic approaches, despite the fact that user led research indicates that service users find a wide variety of non-medical approaches valuable in coping with emotional distress. (Cited in Read et al 2004)

Being prescribed antipsychotic drugs can decrease motivation to seek other pathways to recovery. It is not only the soporific effect on mental functioning that prevents people from thinking about psychosocial explanations for their troubled states of mind, it is also the implicit message swallowed with the pill that there is something medically wrong with you (Ross & Read 2004).

A confused and worrying picture exists about the efficacy and safety of psychotropic drugs. If we take antipsychotic drugs as an example, they do not work for everybody, and there are some studies that suggest that their efficacy in preventing relapse may be limited to as low as one third of clients taking the drug, even when optimal adherence to the medication regime is maintained (Kinderman & Cooke 2000). Yet frequently these drugs, sometimes in combination, continue to be prescribed for individuals, despite the absence of a therapeutic response, even though there is good evidence that if a person fails to respond to one antipsychotic drug they will fail to respond to others (Bentall 2003). Despite claims to the contrary, the newer so-called atypical antipsychotic drugs are no more effective or better tolerated than conventional drugs (Geddes et al 2000). Clearly, people who do not benefit from medication would benefit from drug free strategies for managing symptoms, yet to date such an alternative is not widely available in mental health services.

If the efficacy of these drugs is questionable, then the side-effects are even more concerning. There are a number of distressing side-effects with both conventional and atypical drugs. The older antipsychotic drugs produce extrapyramidal side-effects which include akathisia, tremor, rigidity, dystonia, oculogyric crisis and tardive dyskinesia. This latter disability, involving the involuntary movement of the mouth and tongue, has a prevalence rate among people on conventional antipsychotic drugs of 30% (Llorca et al 2002) and is irreversible in 75% of cases (Hill 1986). Added to this are various anticholinergic effects such as blurred vision, dry mouth and constipation. Also common are weight gain, sexual dysfunction, lethargy and neuroleptic dysphoria – a form of depressive apathy. In a small number of cases, more serious, life-threatening side-effects occur such as agranulocytosis, neuroleptic malignant syndrome and heart failure. While more extensive independent research is needed, there is emerging evidence that prolonged use of antipsychotic drugs may cause a permanent impairment of mental functioning (Breggin 1993). Even the most cursory look at the side-effect profile of antipsychotic medication offers an explanation as to why so many people discontinue taking them.

In a graphic description of his experience of side-effects, Chadwick (1997) states:

with akathisia there is never any peace from the insistent urge to move, be it to rock backwards and forwards in a chair, shuffle around the ward, kneel and huddle in a chair or go for a walk. It is like tinnitus of the body; there is never a moment of inner silence. I remember one day staring into a mirror on Ward 3. My eyeballs were bulging, my skin was greasy and grainy, my hair like rats' tails. I was stiffened and troubled by constipation and simultaneously racked by akathisia. I looked like everybody's image of a mental patient – but it was entirely the medication effect. (p. 50)

Despite this distressing experience and his psychotherapeutic orientation, Chadwick goes on to discuss how low-dose antipsychotic medication has played an important role in his recovery, alongside spiritual, psychosocial and cognitive behavioural approaches.

So to what extent can medication offer a way to recovery? As someone who has used medication at various points in my life I would say that it can provide relief from the relentlessness of troubled thoughts and feelings of despair. It can create a 'breathing space' to regain some resilience and rationality – a point from which deeper healing can be sought or an alternative recovery strategy put in place. Many people would take an opposing view. Chamberlin (1999), in a discourse on non-compliance, argues that for her drugs were part of the problem rather than the solution and simply made her 'fat, lethargic and unable to think or remember'. She argues that while drugs work for some people, for others, including herself, it is 'only when we clear ourselves of all psychiatric drugs that we begin to find the road to recovery'.

Service users' reflections on medication (cited in Mental Health Foundation 1997)

'The drug blocks out most of the voices and delusions and keeps my mood stable'

'The dosages depressed me and made me feel my motivation, ideas and whole autonomy was being forcibly removed'

'Medication is a necessary evil as I have little to fall back on otherwise. The medication stops the psychotic symptoms (or has in the past)'

'Although helpful, on the high dose it took away my psychic awareness and also deadened me emotionally leaving me de-motivated and I spent three years mostly sleeping and watching TV'

'With major tranquillisers I feel as if I'm in a trance. I don't feel like myself. They make me quite paranoid'

There is always a balance sheet to be drawn up when making a decision about whether to take medication, particularly long term, and a willingness on the part of mental health professionals to engage in a collaborative dialogue about the pros and cons of medication can be invaluable (Box 3.6). It can be difficult for some people, particularly in the early stages of recovery, to marshal their thoughts about taking medication, with the result that they end up being passive recipients of medication rather than active participants in making an informed choice. Deegan (1999) suggests some useful strategies to enable people to become active participants in their decision about whether to include medication as part of their recovery plan (Box 3.7).

Box 3.6

Balance sheet for reviewing medication use

Pros
- Relief from symptoms
- Prevention of relapse
- Spending less time in hospital
- Improvement in social functioning
- Improvement in mental functioning
- Achievement of personal goals
- Fits an acceptable medical rationale of mental health problems
- Use medication alongside other recovery resources
- Can take the minimum therapeutic dose
- Choosing to use medication as part of recovery/ not simply taking it

Cons
- It provides no relief from symptoms or relapses
- Experience of side-effects
- Risk of long-term side-effects
- Problems withdrawing from medication
- Experience of dysphoria
- Availability of evidence-based alternatives to drug treatment
- Stigma of taking medication/undermining of positive self-image
- Militates against understanding the origins and meaning of distress
- Militates against use of alternative coping strategies
- Feeling of being coerced into taking medication

Box 3.7

Thinking about medication

Strategy 1: Learn to think differently about medication
- Medication is not a panacea. Medication alone will not make a person better – you cannot sit back and wait to recover. Recovery means taking an active stance towards the problems and challenges of life.
- Medication is only one facet of a recovery strategy – exercise, spiritual practice, creativity, work, communion with the natural world, complementary therapies, supportive personal relationships and friendships can be equally important.
- There is moral neutrality in the act of using prescribed medication – it is neither good nor bad, right nor wrong. The decision to use effective medication within the recovery process as a way of realising personal goals may reflect thoughtful expediency.

- Other interventions such as cognitive behavioural therapy can be helpful in alleviating distress symptoms and preventing relapse. Learning these strategies can eliminate or reduce the need for medication.

- Drugs are never problem-free. There is always a cost/benefit analysis to be done before using medication – positive outcomes in terms of the reduction of disabling and distressing symptoms versus adverse drug reactions.

Strategy 2: Learn to think differently about yourself

- Each individual is the expert on his or her own experience and it is important to trust that experience. Keeping a diary of your responses to medication, both helpful and adverse, can help in finding the most effective drug for you.

- Never attribute all improvement to medication. Look at the things you have done to facilitate and maintain your recovery.

- Assert your right to question mental health professionals about new or current medication. 'Is it worth continuing to take this medication?' 'Are there alternatives to medication?' 'Are there other drugs worth trying?' 'Is this the lowest therapeutic dose I can take?' 'How will I know if this medication is working for me?' 'How long will it take to work?' 'What are the common side-effects of this medication?' 'What are the more serious side-effects of this medication?' 'How often do they occur?' 'How difficult is it to withdraw from this medication?' 'Have any studies been done of the long-term effects of this drug?' 'Have any studies been done on the effects of drug combinations?' 'Could my need for medication have changed over time?' 'What would be the risks of stopping my medication and how can those risks be minimised?' 'Can people recover from the experience of psychosis without medication?' These are all valid questions to which you should expect a satisfactory answer.

- A planned withdrawal from medication should include alternative coping strategies, an awareness of the withdrawal syndrome; an awareness of early signs of relapse and contingency plans for dealing with any crisis, which may or may not include the resumption of medication.

Strategy 3: Learn to think differently about the way you relate to mental health professionals

- Psychiatrists are the acknowledged experts on psychotropic medication but they may be biologically biased and not give you a balanced view of the likely causes of your distress experience and the recovery options. Always ask about alternative treatment modalities.

- It is not wise to assume that your psychiatrist has a thorough knowledge of your treatment history. They may not be aware of the different drugs and drug combinations you have used over the years. It can be helpful to compile and keep your own record of this.

- Psychiatrists and general practitioners are not immune from the influence of the multinational pharmaceutical companies. While the humanitarian quest to discover chemical agents that relieve human suffering is laudable, there is a dark underbelly to 'Big Pharma'. The profit motive drives the industry into questionable ethical practices such as the publication of selected research studies that portray their product in the most favourable light. It is wise to assume that no drug is as efficacious or as 'clean' as it is said to be.

- Be prepared to set the agenda for your meetings with mental health professionals. If you want to discuss specific medication issues or alternative strategies, say so at the beginning of the meeting.

- Write down your questions and observations and bring them with you to meetings. Preparing in this way can help you hold on to your power and develop a more collaborative way of relating to mental health professionals.
- Bring a friend or advocate with you who can support you in articulating your concerns, questions and points of view. They can also remind you of what was said during the meeting.
- Sometimes it can be helpful to take notes or record what is said during a meeting with mental health professionals. Important details can get forgotten because of the anxiety those meetings sometimes cause.

(Adapted from Deegan 1999)

Non-compliance with medication is seldom an irrational act or a decision based on lack of insight. It is much more to do with the negative experiences of 'being on medication'. Even so we have seen the dissemination of an intervention called compliance therapy (Kemp et al 1998), a term that implies that non-adherence to medication is a form of pathology. There can be many reasons for non-adherence and these can only be explored in the context of an open, respectful, non-judgemental dialogue with mental health professionals. We have to free ourselves from the 'medication myths' and start looking at the evidence objectively before we can help people make informed decisions about whether to use medication.

One of these myths is that people in the grip of a psychotic experience need antipsychotic drugs of necessity in order to recover and regain their foothold in the 'real world'. The mythic status of this clinical rationale is exposed by the fact that before the advent of psychotropic drugs in the 1950s many people recovered clinically and socially, particularly if they were cared for in enlightened therapeutic conditions. In more recent times, successful outcomes in the drug-free treatment of schizophrenia have been demonstrated by the Soteria project (Mosher 2004) and replicated in Europe by the Bern project (Ciompi 1997). In addition it has been demonstrated that the outcome for people diagnosed as suffering from schizophrenia is far superior in poorer countries where psychotropic drugs are less readily available compared with richer industrialised societies (Harrison et al 2001).

As Ciompi (1980) sagely put it in a statement that was largely disregarded 25 years ago:

> There is no such thing as a specific course for schizophrenia. Doubtless the potential for improvement of schizophrenia has for a long time been grossly underestimated. What is called the course of schizophrenia more closely resembles a life process open to a great variety of influences of all kinds than an illness with a given course.

For some people the issue of whether or not to take medication is about power. There can be a coercive element to the prescribing and administration of antipsychotic drugs which smacks of social control, an experience reinforced by the 'deadening' effect that these drugs sometimes have. Non-adherence can be seen as way of wresting back some control over one's life. Adherence to prescribed medication requires accepting that there is a neurological dysfunction underlying the distress experience. This is usually conveyed in the form of a diagnosis – schizophrenia or bipolar disorder – along with the information that life-long or at least long-term medication to control symptoms and prevent relapse is advised. The impact of this information on self-image and self-esteem can be considerable and is understandably resisted. For others there is a stigma associated with a reliance on medication or with the more open acknowledgement of mental ill health associated with 'being on medication'. Sometimes the objection to medication is that it suppresses something of the essential being of the individual, and however chaotic and problematic that elemental part of the person is, to have it 'chemically lobotomised' is to feel changed and less alive. If we add to these psychosocial reasons for non-compliance the experience of the unpleasant side-effects discussed above and which are a reality for most people who use psychotropic drugs, it is unsurprising that so many people stop taking medication. Instead of seeing those who are non-compliant as people who refuse treatment, we should see them as individuals who are more discerning in their quest for wellbeing and recovery.

Strengths and the way to recovery

Conventional approaches to care and treatment focus on problems, deficits, disabilities and dysfunction, often defined in relation to the medical model. This view of mental disequilibrium as neuropathology or psychopathology sees problems in living as arising from a malfunction in neurotransmission or psychological complexes – conditions to be treated and cured. If the condition is treatment-resistant and the problems remain despite a battery of therapeutic interventions, the individual joins the cohort of people with severe and enduring mental health problems, people whom psychiatric services have failed to help. But what if we are approaching recovery in the wrong way? How would it be if, instead of giving so much attention to dysfunction, we looked more at people's assets, qualities, skills, accomplishments, aspirations, potentials, interests? How would it be if we looked at what they can do, or aspire to do, at what it is that draws people more fully and confidently into life? So often, people struggling to live in an enduring psychological turmoil become mired in their problem-saturated history, which in some cases submerges their identity altogether. Yet I have not met anyone, even those whose minds and lives have been all but wrecked by psychological turmoil, whose positive attributes and potential to be something more than a victim of misfortune did not shine through.

Attempting to manage someone's vulnerability to recurrent mood swings with lithium and CBT is often a worthwhile intervention but it does not necessarily improve the quality of a person's life or their subjective feeling of wellbeing. However, building on their artistic interest and abilities and helping them to create opportunities for the expression of that interest can pay dividends in terms of increased self-esteem, meaningful activity and social inclusion. Trying to help someone overcome the seemingly intractable apathy, lethargy and dysphoria that has settled on their lives with changes of medication and carefully conceived psychotherapeutic strategies can often be fruitless. What is missing is something to feel aroused, energised and uplifted about. A pathway back into work, training or education that fits with an individual's aspiration and dreams can be more motivating. Having our lives infused with meaning is what enables us to live purposefully and vitally.

In recent years there has been a growing interest in what has become known as positive psychology. Until now clinical psychology has chiefly occupied itself with understanding and resolving distress and disturbance and has virtually neglected positive feeling, whereas this new and exciting field of research is concerned with identifying and maximising what it is that promotes happiness and fulfilment and sustains wellbeing. Martin Seligman, a leading figure in the positive psychology movement, argues that what underpins *authentic happiness* is the expression of our *core values and signature strengths* in our everyday lives (Seligman 2002). By core values he means those virtues that have been universally endorsed by the world religions and schools of philosophy, namely wisdom and knowledge, courage, love and compassion, justice, moderation, spirituality and transcendence. Our signature strengths are those traits that characterise our behaviour through which we express these core values. So, for example, kindness and generosity might be a characteristic trait which expresses the core values of love and compassion; similarly, integrity, honesty and genuineness display moral courage; and playfulness and humour or the appreciation of beauty communicate our transcendent nature. Seligman believes that we all have a unique personal profile of signature strengths and the more integrated they are into our way of being in the world, the greater our sense of happiness and wellbeing. Identifying with this hypothesis is not difficult – most of us recognise that we feel good when we have done something honourable or loving, have satisfied our wide-eyed curiosity about something previously little understood, or shown moderation in response to some self-gratifying urge. It seems to me that positive psychology offers mental health practitioners a potentially powerful focus for recovery work through working alongside clients helping them to identify and find ways of expressing more of their signature strengths in everyday life.

The strengths approach to mental health care offers a strong philosophical basis for practice and has a growing evidence base to support its efficacy (Barry et al 2003). With its emphasis on the realisation of potentials and aspirations and the fulfilment of needs, it is at the heart of recovery (Box 3.8). The model does not deny the existence of the psychological and social problems which can have a devastating impact on people's lives but attempts to help people live and live well, sometimes in spite of those continuing vulnerabilities. If we can help people identify their goals and recognise their strengths and resources, if we can believe in the ability of everyone to grow and change and be a supportive presence to people in that process, then problems that seemed insurmountable become less so. Professor Charles Rapp, the originator of the strengths approach, puts it this way: the strengths model sets out 'to assist consumers in identifying, securing and sustaining a range of resources – both environmental and personal needed to live, play and work in a normally interdependent way in the community' (Rapp 1998). This moves the work of practitioners away from problem solving towards a more facilitative role, a role that is concerned with the client's personal growth and social inclusion.

Many of us spend our lives 'waiting for Godot' – waiting for that moment when life will miraculously change for us and we will leave the stultifying disappointment of our spoilt lives and find ourselves on those sun-filled uplands fulfilling our true destiny. What we fail to be fully cognisant of is that life is here and now – this is it – and no one but ourselves has the responsibility or the will to change it. Yet we wait for that something or someone who will sprinkle fairy dust on our lives and in waiting fail to seize the moment to set off in the direction of a life well lived. The strengths approach is an exhortation to set off on the road to recovery, where we will realise more of our potential and find more of the life satisfactions we seek.

Box 3.8

Strength-based principles

- The focus of the helping process is on service users' strengths, interests, abilities and capabilities, not upon their deficits, weaknesses, problems.
- All service users have the capacity to learn, grow and change.
- The service user–practitioner relationship becomes a collaborative partnership.
- The service user is the director of the helping process.
- Continuity and acceptance are essential foundations for promoting recovery.
- The helping process takes on an outreach perspective.
- The local neighbourhood is viewed as a source of potential resources rather than as an obstacle. Natural neighbourhood resources should be considered before segregated mental health services.

(Morgan 2004)

It is not enough to pay lip service to this way of working. We have to weave it into the very fabric of our practice, make it the *raison d'être* of our service. Most service users are tired of their problem-saturated lives, tired of stigmatising psychiatric labels, of being defined by past disabilities, failures, inadequacies and misdemeanours. Most of all they are tired of being undermined and infantilised by 'expert'-led care. They are ready for something different. It can be hope inspiring and strengthening to have your positive attributes, potentials and aspirations acknowledged and at the centre of your care plan. It can be empowering to be approached in a truly collaborative way, to feel that you have the freedom and the responsibility to take decisions about your care and treatment and about your life. It is important that mental health workers fully embrace the implications of this and intervene in a way that countermands the client's self-determination only when there is clear risk to the safety or welfare of that person and/or others.

The perception of someone using mental health services viewed from the strengths perspective is very different from that of a person seen from a problem-orientated viewpoint, the focus being on the resources a person has (or that are available to them in their community) which can be utilised to help them move towards a life with a measure of the joy and satisfaction we all seek. It is about defining goals: 'What are the things that give you a sense satisfaction and pleasure in your life?' 'What is it that gives a sense of meaning and purpose to your life?' Responding to these questions can be hard, particularly when one's life has been impoverished and marginalised for some time. Nevertheless, in a continuing dialogue which is strengths-focused, aspects of life that bring pleasure and purpose emerge (Fig. 3.3).

Self Enquiry Box

You may like to explore this strengths evaluation (Fig. 3.3) yourself before adapting it for use with clients. The evaluation scale is simply a tool for stimulating and structuring a discussion around strengths and values in the domains of everyday life. Each domain can be teased out to give it more specificity, for example the relationship domain includes personal, family, friends, workmates, neighbours. Identifying values in everyday life may be more difficult and has to be worked at, but it is a worthwhile task given that there is increasing evidence that the expression of our core values in the domains of life experience equates with happiness and wellbeing. Similarly, finding meaning and purpose is strongly linked with a sense of fulfilment and wellbeing. Meaning and purpose may be faith based or linked to family relationships, duties and responsibilities. They may be found in the work we choose to do, through social action for the greater good, in living an ethical life, actualising our potentials as human beings or expressing our creativity.

It is not that the problematic elements in a person's life are ignored – of course we are concerned with what is going on and going wrong – but the emphasis is placed on what needs to happen for life to be more sustaining, less problematic; what the resources are on which a person can draw to make that a reality. This can be enormously empowering and inspiring, tipping the balance away from expert-led care and service-based resources and towards self-efficacy and community-based resources. We have to stop defining people by their vulnerabilities and problem-saturated lives and start seeing their positive attributes, achievements and aspirations. Simply looking at the recovery journeys of the people who have generously shared their stories in this book shows that what has prompted and sustained their recovery is not any particular therapeutic intervention but the will and resourcefulness of the individuals concerned. For one contributor it was trusting the wisdom of the inner voice to guide his recovery; cleansing the body and mind of toxic influences to allow self-healing to take place and supporting that process further by using holistic therapies.

Domains of experience

Relationships

How satisfied am I with the interpersonal dimension of my life?

Not satisfied   Very satisfied

Occupation

How satisfied am I with my job/voluntary work/training/education/main daytime activity?

Not satisfied   Very satisfied

Leisure

How satisfied am I with the way I spend my leisure time?

Not satisfied   Very satisfied

Community

How satisfied am I with my social/cultural/political expression of citizenship?

Not satisfied   Very satisfied

Economic

How satisfied am I with the way I manage my personal finances?

Not satisfied   Very satisfied

Home

How satisfied am I with my living space?

Not satisfied   Very satisfied

Spirituality

How satisfied am I with the spiritual/religious/transcendent dimension of my life?

Not satisfied   Very satisfied

Sexuality

How satisfied am I with the way I express my sexuality?

Not satisfied   Very satisfied

Health and wellbeing

How satisfied am I with the way I manage my mental/physical health?

Not satisfied   Very satisfied

Figure 3.3 ● Strengths and values evaluation.

Key questions
- What skills, qualities, accomplishments, resources have I utilised in achieving that degree of satisfaction?
- What would be present in my life that's not there now, if I were to move one degree further towards being very satisfied in that domain?
- What additional resources, personal or community, would I need to access to achieve that?
- What gives my life purpose and meaning?
- Am I able to give that purpose and meaning centrality in the domains of experience my life encompasses?
- What values are important to me in the way I live my life, e.g. honesty, love, kindness, forgiveness, creativity, learning, humour, beauty, self-control, perseverance, integrity, community, zest, fairness, calm?
- Do I express those values in the domains of experience my life encompasses?

Figure 3.3 ● Continued.

For another, it was stepping away from a life as a 'career patient' and using her compassion and experience to secure meaningful employment caring for others. A third contributor was able to release her imprisoned self through keeping a journal and writing poetry. In every case it was the mobilisation of inner strengths and resources that precipitated and sustained the recovery journey.

During the asylum period, mental hospitals were virtually self-sufficient communities, segregated from the host community. It is a sad fact that moving mental health care out from the institution has not led to a real experience of social inclusion for people with continuing mental health problems. In part, this is because many day care resources, sited in and around urban centres, create asylums in miniature which do not provide the impetus for people to access community facilities and include themselves more fully in mainstream life. In helping clients to meet their identified needs and realise personal goals, we should think of the community in which they live as a potential resource and not as some hinterland that is impossible or difficult to traverse. I am not saying that for many people there are not significant barriers to be overcome, of course there are, but surely we should be working with people to overcome these and claim their right to full citizenship rather than consigning them to 'sanctuaries for the vulnerable'?

Recovery can be a long-term project. People who have experienced continuing mental health problems over many years are often adrift in a tempestuous internal world and seem to have lost the means to navigate to calmer waters. Others have built up strong defences against personal and social change, doggedly maintaining the status quo of their lives at a low level of social and mental functioning, not daring, as Samuel Beckett put it, to 'fail again and fail better'. Some continue to use drugs and alcohol as self-medication or as lifestyle choices, despite their deleterious effect on their mental health. Many, having given up hope of the possibility of any other life, have all but surrendered to hopelessness, helplessness and passivity. Others meet their emotional needs through the sick role, clinging on to their symptoms to legitimise the emotional comfort they get from others. So pervasive are their abandonment anxieties that any recovery work is likely to be sabotaged.

Whatever the dynamic that acts as a barrier to recovery, overcoming it is likely to be a protracted process. Services similarly need to be thought of as long term to provide the continuity people need in order to begin and sustain their recovery journey. How frustrating and demoralising it must be to be regularly faced with unfamiliar workers who may not know where the client is on their journey and may relate more to their history than their current life situation. Continuity can be achieved in services such as assertive outreach where there is a long-term commitment to clients and a team approach underpins individual case management. The team holds collective responsibility for the work with clients and it is likely that clients will know and be known by some if not all members of the team.

Assertive outreach

The strengths approach is being widely adopted as a philosophical basis for practice by assertive outreach (AO) teams (Ryan & Morgan 2004). There has always been some unease about the term 'assertive' because of the connotation of an authoritarian, intrusive approach to care. To my mind it is a perfect adjective to describe the nature of outreach work. To be assertive is to be respectful of others' rights and needs while at the same time having regard for one's own. Enshrined within the term is a belief in the essential worth of oneself and others and in relating to others as equals. Assertiveness is not about the dominance of one person over another; it is about collaboration.

AO is now well established in Britain with over 200 teams in place. It is an evolving service, rooted in a person-centred recovery model. The remit of AO is to engage and work with people who experience severe mental health problems and have complex needs, in particular those people who constitute a high risk and those who are reluctant to engage with mental health services or, conversely and more pertinently, those with whom conventional mental health services find it difficult to engage (Box 3.9).

In a review of the evidence for AO, Ryan & Morgan (2004) highlight a discrepancy between the more positive outcomes documented in the international literature and the British experience. The evidence from UK studies for the efficacy of AO in preventing hospitalisation, reducing risk and symptomatology is not conclusive. However, studies that have evaluated engagement with services, quality of life and service user and carer satisfaction with AO services demonstrate a strongly positive outcome (Ryan et al 1999; Grayley-Wetherell & Morgan 2001). It is difficult to account for this discrepancy between international studies and the UK experience. Perhaps in many teams fidelity to the AO model is not maintained or training in the approach inadequate. Statistics, however, never tell the whole story and while admission rates for AO clients may have remained unchanged, bed days are likely to have been reduced and AO admissions are often planned as part of the client's proactive crisis management plan.

Positive risk-taking is the AO way. Recovery cannot be nurtured in the context of defensive practice. To grow and change in adaptive ways people need freedom

74

Box 3.9

Non-engagement issues

- Negative experiences of mental health workers and the psychiatric system
- An understanding of the distress experience which differs from that of mental health professionals
- Therapeutic pessimism of mental health professionals
- Mental health services have little to offer that is experienced as helpful
- Fear of the legal power of mental health services
- Fear of the loss of sovereignty over one's life
- See referral to mental health services as a hallmark of inadequacy, failure or weakness
- Threat to identity posed by the mythology of 'madness'
- Fear of being labelled, stigmatised or discriminated against
- Sexism, racism and homophobia of mental health workers
- Continuity of workers or services is lacking
- Availability and accessibility of workers is limited
- Fear of intimacy or of being vulnerable
- Denial of mental health problems
- Transference and counter-transference issues

from those aspects of psychiatric practice that would manacle the mind and institutionalise a life. In the engagement process a narrow focus on symptoms can be disadvantageous. A person's symptomatology needs to be accepted and tolerated to allow a person-centred relationship to flourish. Symptom escalation is always likely to happen as clients begin their recovery journey and seek to engage more fully in life, but this can be seen as a further opportunity for people to learn about themselves, about their early signs of relapse, about triggers and about how to manage the intensification of their symptoms so that a state of psychological overwhelm does not continue to be the outcome. Positive gains can emerge out of the creative management of crisis, such as self-awareness and personal responsibility, the cornerstones of recovery.

AO is not just about engagement; this is simply a prerequisite for a long-term commitment to a person's recovery – recovery of a quality of life, a life that is less problematic and more fulfilling, a recovery based on more than the maintenance of a symptom-free life. What is clear is that many people who are reluctant to engage with services find in the person-centred approach of AO workers a basis of trust that leads to a deepening working alliance that is in itself a catalyst for positive change.

Recovery, as we have seen, can be a long-term project. It follows that recovery teams need to sustain their own wellbeing if the creative energy and commitment of staff are to be maintained. In my own service, the emotional and practical burden of the work is carried by the team. This can be a difficult mindset on which to base practice but, once assimilated, the 'therapeutic ego' and the 'must cope' mentality dissolve and the strengths and creativity of the whole team become more visible and available to the client. Consequently staff stress and burnout – endemic in long-term psychiatric work – diminish.

As Morgan rightly argues, a strengths philosophy should permeate the organisational culture of mental health services and not be seen simply as a therapeutic stance. Do we value the skills, abilities, qualities and potentials of colleagues enough? Are mental health workers entrusted with the responsibility for their own development as professionals and given the support to realise those aspirations? Is the working environment one that is empowering and capable of encouraging growth; one that sustains the wellbeing, creativity and commitment of the team? Is the leadership style strongly facilitative? These are crucial questions, as organisational systems which do not enshrine these values are hardly likely to produce a culture within which recovery-orientated practice can flourish.

Whatever direction 'the way' takes, it is essentially about growth and change. A common experience for people who have experienced long periods of distress which may have often erupted in their late teens and continued through early adult life is that they have missed out on considerable developmental experience. Their lives may have become too reclusive, too preoccupied with unusual mental phenomena, too overwhelmed by depressive feelings and thoughts, too threatened by paranoid anxieties, too often 'out of it' on street drugs, to participate in life. Many young people who enter the psychiatric system feel too perplexed and disturbed by their experience, too discouraged and helpless to say yes to life, or too numb or fatigued as the result of prescribed medication to feel fully alive. Family relationships or professional relationships in which the quest for autonomy, responsibility and independence may have been stifled can exacerbate this. When we consider the stigma and discrimination people with a psychiatric history face, we can begin to see what a formidable challenge it can be for young men and women to reclaim a place for themselves in society. The coalescence of all the negative factors in the life of an individual robs them of enormous amount of developmental experience and after years of struggling with disabling distress, there can be a significant developmental lag to be overcome in the recovery journey.

A great deal of building up needs to take place, of self-acceptance, self-esteem, self-confidence, without which the recovery journey will not be possible (Coleman 1999). Coleman makes the salient observation, based on his own recovery experience, that you need to 'give up being ill so you can start being recovered'. This means beginning to take some responsibility for your life, claiming your rights to full citizenship. It means finding constructive, socially valued ways of being occupied, seeking friendships and establishing personal relationships, making a home of your own. These are not simply the social hallmarks of adulthood, they are the looms on which the mantle of growth and maturity is woven. It can be a difficult and painful process. There can be rejections, disappointments and failures but this is part of the living learning experience of everyone. For some people the barriers can seem insurmountable but, to use a line from a civil rights song, the important thing is to 'keep your eye on the prize, hold on, hold on'.

The return

Quest: to return from the journey stronger and wiser

The return to sanity and wellbeing is a journey of many months, sometimes many years; it is not so much a completion point in our developmental history as a point when we return to the place from which we started, seeing it and ourselves clearly for perhaps the first time. We will have come to know our strengths and weaknesses, our qualities and our fallibilities. We will accept ourselves with all our imperfections, failures and triumphs with generous self-regard, humility and good humour. We will have learned how to live, how to say yes to life. We are not the same person who set out on the hero's journey. To return to that previous incarnation and to the life that was lived then would be to occupy the same perilous position. We are still vulnerable – human beings are vulnerable – but we now recognise our personal power. It seems to me that recovery really is a *return to our senses:* we return from a journey through madness with a much heightened sense of what it means to be human and have more compassion and joy and somehow seem more connected to others and the world at large.

The recovery journey is never straightforward: our wellbeing and equanimity are always likely to be threatened by the challenges and adversities that are part of life. Often there are specific stressors to which we are particularly sensitive that will trigger a return of a distressed and troubled state of mind. Becoming familiar with our relapse signature and being aware of and responsive to these early signs that have in the past heralded a reoccurrence of disturbed feelings, thoughts and behaviour opens up the possibility of taking early restorative action.

But we should not think of the return of our distress as a failure, weakness or inadequacy. We should not give up the recovery journey and surrender our life to overwhelming distress; re-entering the realms of 'madness' is one of the trials along the way to healing. It is at times like these that one must find the courage and fortitude to continue the search for the epiphany that lies at the heart of our madness. Every journey into the outer reaches of our psyches is an opportunity to discover the meaning of our disturbed state of mind and to return with greater self-knowledge and self-regard – a potentially transforming and strengthening experience (Breggin 1997). Caplan (1964) in his seminal work on crisis theory proposed that a crisis should be seen as a potential turning point, that although it may be a painful and disorganising experience it is also an opportunity to learn something helpful about our lives and ourselves. Deegan (1993), in discussing her own recovery from severe mental illness, is passionate in stressing the need to regard relapse episodes as breaking out or breaking through: 'It may mean I'm breaking out of some prison or fear filled place where I have been trapped inside myself. It may mean I'm breaking through into a different way of being' (p. 10).

Of course this is not easy. Many people struggle for years with recurrent disturbing, distressing experiences before some resolution takes place. Some people regard themselves as being *in recovery* rather than recovered. This suggests that healing may never be complete, that half-healed wounds may reopen. The task that faces people as they travel along the recovery road is to become 'experts' at actively managing their mental health and sustaining their sense of wellbeing. Deegan regards her own recovery as a process rather than a destination, something that has to be worked at every day:

> *To me recovery means staying in the driver's seat of my life. I don't let my illness run me. Over the years I've worked hard at being an expert in my own self-care. For me being in recovery doesn't mean just taking medication which is a passive stance, rather, I use medication as part of my recovery process. In the same way I don't just go to the hospital, rather I use the hospital when I need to. I use medication, therapy, self-help strategies, mutual support groups, friends, my relationship with God, work, exercise, spending time with nature – all of these measures help me remain whole and healthy even though I have a disability. (p. 10)*

In reflecting on the recovery process as a heroic journey I am not indulging in metaphorical games: it can be long, it can be arduous and challenging, but ultimately transformative (Fig. 3.4). It is heroic! It can be enormously difficult to start and continue on that journey. As we have seen, one third of people that are diagnosed with a severe mental health problem struggle to recover. They spend much of their life in the grip of uncontainable troubling thoughts, feelings and perceptions or caught up in pervasive dysphoria and apathy and continue to live marginalised lives with recurrent, sometimes extended periods of time in hospital. I do not believe it has to be this way. There is no evidence of an innate susceptibility to chronicity in psychosis (Harrison et al 2001).

So why is that some people, despite the best efforts of family, friends and services, cannot stay free of disturbing mental intrusions for long, cannot maintain a state of emotional balance, cannot find an island of calm, and seem forever adrift in a sea of agitated fearfulness, all of which makes it hard to sustain a reasonable level of wellbeing. In charting the hero's journey we have come across a number of factors that might be part of this state of affairs: the sealed off way of coping; the stasis and passivity that settle on a person's life; a pervasive sense of powerlessness; the unresolved grief; the continuing use of street drugs and alcohol; social marginalisation; the lack of a therapeutic response to optimal medication; the absence of alternative interventions; a lack of meaning and purpose in life; the eclipse of someone's identity, along with their strengths and potentials, by a continuing mental health problem; the seduction of madness; the developmental gap; and a family life that is not conducive to growth and recovery.

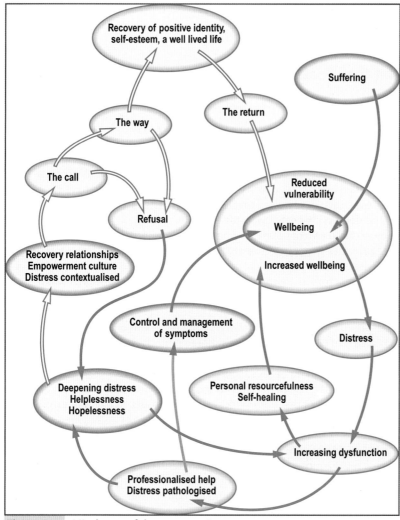

Figure 3.4 ● Mind map of the recovery journey.

All of these factors can conspire to create obstacles on someone's road to recovery. In the last analysis perhaps it all comes down to needing something or someone to recover for. It is those dreams, aspirations, expectations we have of our future that draw us on into life. If our dreams are shattered, as they undoubtedly can be by a severe mental health problem, then it is difficult to rebuild those towering hopes and we find ourselves in a bleak place where once stood the edifice of our life. Those of us who are professionally entrusted to be companions to people on their road to recovery, as well as families, friends – all of us – have to hold to the belief that life can be less troubled, less problematic, more fulfilling. There is no magic fix that we can prescribe but there is a transformative power in believing in someone, in their potential to become something more, in their capacity to heal and recover.

The metal that floats – a personal reflection on recovery

John McCloud

My first experience of depression was on a skiing holiday a few weeks after my fifteenth birthday. The following autumn, in 1973, I started sixth form, and within a few days of arriving back at boarding school I was anxious, my stomach felt empty, I started to wake about four or five in the morning and not get back to sleep. However, I only really had one genuine worry, which was whether I should have chosen to do Latin 'A' level. Each day I hoped that I would wake the next day feeling better, and I didn't. The depression probably lasted a month.

I'd already endured two depressions when in the autumn of 1974 I became manic. The headmaster wrote to my parents that if I didn't see a psychiatrist, or at least the family doctor, I would be expelled.

This development forced me to think about my life more analytically. I was on an English 'A' level course, and I'd come across the concept of manic depression in an introduction to John Clare's poetry and also in an obscure critique of Hamlet. Looking back through my diaries I'd known that my self-confidence gyrated wildly and I now realised that I had for some time suffered periods of depression followed by periods of normalcy and then elation. Stumbling across my diagnosis in this way was on the one hand daunting because there was the possibility of experiencing these mood swings for the rest of my life, but the up-side was that I was sharing a diagnosis with my heroes of that time, writers and composers. As a teenager already somewhat off course, this revelation provided me with a kind of instant identity.

A considerable amount of the anxiety I was feeling when depressed was caused by the fact that I could not understand what was happening to me. The first depression after I knew my diagnosis felt qualitatively different. I didn't have to worry what was causing it. Similarly, I didn't worry about whether I was going to wake up feeling the same way the next day, as this was beyond my control and, more importantly, the depression would inevitably come to an end, as it was only part of the cycle. The important consideration was how best to cope with the depression. During my sixth form years, I was often either too depressed to work or too elated to want to work. I was under pressure, mostly from myself, to rescue the situation and not flunk my 'A' levels. In the Easter holidays before my exams, my revision and my first major breakdown melded into one.

I remember the psychiatrist appealing to me to trust him. If you trust your psychiatrist, however, it is possible that he remains the 'expert', and you remain a passive patient. Much better to find out as much about your illness as possible, to see if the diagnosis fits your symptoms and find out how best to deal with your illness! In my case the first two psychiatrists who treated me made mistakes. The psychiatrist who diagnosed me with manic depression changed his mind, without explicit explanation, and prescribed me Depixol, an antipsychotic drug, which I was on for a couple of years, and was, in retrospect, pointless. The second psychiatrist made mistakes for ideological reasons. He appeared to believe that there was no such thing as mental illness, and consequently didn't believe in diagnosis, or any drug treatment. As a result, instead of being prescribed lithium, I was led on a futile six year psychotherapeutic journey of self-discovery and found myself shuttling between mental hospital and therapeutic community.

When in hospital I was liberally dosed with Largactil, haloperidol and Valium to contain my highs, as well as receiving ECT. My manic depression was at its worst between the ages of 18 and 24, depressions and highs lasting six months or more. Being bludgeoned with 1950s medication and half-baked 1970s ideas simply allowed me to be a manic depressive to the full. The strategy of avoiding diagnosis didn't work, with my parents most of all having to deal with the fall out. Although my relationship with my parents was severely strained by my manic episodes, the biggest factor in my favour during these years was, I think, parental support. For example, when I was 20 and living in London in a therapeutic hostel and severely depressed, my parents allowed me to come home. I don't know how I would have coped, and many have to, if I had been totally cut off from my family in those years.

It wasn't until I was 24 and had fallen under the jurisdiction of another psychiatrist that I was prescribed and took lithium for long enough to make a difference. My social worker got me into a college of further education to do two 'A' levels and into a county run residential hostel on the agreement that I was left to get on with the course. This was the first time that the arrangements made for me by my social worker and my own wishes really coincided. At this time, the autumn of 1982, I was mildly depressed, but in a way that allowed me to work. After a few weeks at college my history lecturer suggested I apply to university, which I did. I had a relapse when I first started my degree, and then I didn't have another relapse for four and a half years, during which time I'd finished my degree, done an MA, and was some way through a postgraduate teaching course. I put this down to being on the right dose of lithium, and having a sense of purpose.

Being on lithium brought to an end the long, sometimes enjoyable highs (before they got out of hand) that I'd had in my late teens and early twenties. But it seems to me possible that the denied high or low as a result of being on lithium can sometimes come out in different ways. In my case I was increasingly troubled by voices, which I was probably imagining, but nevertheless could appear to have a life of their own. I was somewhat released from this purgatory of voices, when, at the beginning of 1988, I had a manic episode and was admitted to a mental hospital on a Sunday morning. This episode blighted my teaching career, because the price of being allowed to finish the teaching course was having the term 'hypomania' on my reference from the college. As I understand it, hypomania means a milder form of manic excitement, but I suspect to laity it could mean the complete opposite of everything we hold dear in civilisation. I managed to get a temporary teaching post in my home county after finishing the postgraduate certificate in education, but despite making several applications and teaching competently and reliably as a supply teacher, I was never offered a permanent post. To my mind the discrimination by the Local Education Authority was completely clear cut – the term hypomania made 100% of the difference.

There is clearly a difference, as well as a link, between recovery and realising one's potential. While I feel I have largely recovered from manic depression, I don't think I realised my potential in my career. If I had realised my potential as an employed teacher, I think I would have almost forgotten that I was, or am, a manic depressive. The LEA's decision not to employ me on health grounds had been without any access to my medical records, or doctors that might have known me, and must have been based purely on the two or three sentences that accompanied my original reference. I appealed against this decision, lost my appeal and as a result could no longer teach in schools in a temporary or permanent capacity.

After leaving teaching, I worked for a small publishing company for five years. There was then a period of several more years without episodes, during which time a psychiatrist in the outpatient department started to discuss with me ways of identifying the high earlier, to shorten the treatment time. This was the most concerted effort I'd experienced to develop my expertise in managing my aberrant mood. The agreed early warning signs were: poor sleep; laughing; mind racing; feeling different; harking back to previous highs; entering a fantasy world and becoming obsessed by certain trains of thought. The psychiatrist had a bottle of haloperidol made up with instructions to be 'taken after sleep disturbed for two nights accompanied by active thinking'. 'Harking back to previous highs' is the phrase that always sticks in my mind, and that I find most useful. It identifies a process that invariably happens when going high, and not at other times, and signals this as a warning. It is like a mental replay of the highs of my late teens and early twenties and it makes me seriously question the wisdom of such a reenactment in the context of my present life.

Around this time, there also seems to have been an improvement in the drugs available to curb a high. I had always found the side-effects of haloperidol crippling; you couldn't possibly function on it so my decision to take the drug was often delayed, but the delay made the situation worse. A further incentive for me to intervene early is that over the last few years I've got more cowardly about the side-effects of the drugs I might be given. Additionally, if you are very high, coming down from the high itself and getting that first bit of sleep, is also frightening.

Now, if necessary, I take risperidone, and I take even a shortened night's sleep as being a possible sign of deterioration. Sometimes worries take a slightly paranoid turn, and if that then tips over into the escalating high thought train I would have to think about taking risperidone. Currently, I am getting through about seven 1 mg tablets a year. The side-effects are sufficiently obvious to mean that I miss a couple of days work. I also occasionally take sleeping tablets, as I can be so obsessive that it keeps me awake, but I probably take less than five of these a year. I am still taking the lithium. However, I wouldn't want these very low doses to be seen as just a testament to my skills of self-managing manic depression, but more importantly as the extent to which early onset manic depression can subside in later life of its own accord.

In 1991 I met Alison, and as a result a few years later I had the confidence to become self-employed. We are now married and have two children, currently aged five and seven. My family life is fundamental to my happiness and sense of wellbeing and to my sense of self-worth. My wife is someone I can trust, and she doesn't allow me to deny my symptoms. As symptoms rock the boat, I often initially deny that I am experiencing them.

Since 1991, I have had three hospital admissions, one in 1996, and two in 1999. The second admission in 1999 was delayed by a couple of days because the GP couldn't get a hospital bed in this area. By the time I was admitted two days later I was so paranoid and terrified that I ran away from the hospital almost as soon as I'd arrived, and recovery was very protracted. Since then I've found that early intervention, described above, works a lot better, and keeps the time that I am 'away' down to a couple of days.

I think manic depression is something you are born with; a form of neurological susceptibility. It seems to me that when manic depressives talk about it they sometimes confuse causes with triggers. For me, the trigger for manic depression to show itself was the physical changes of adolescence and I have no doubt that whatever environment I had been in, manic depression would still have made its appearance. For this reason, I believe that soul searching and looking for causes in your childhood or background is irrelevant. Childhood experience might make you more or less cautious or more or less fearful of rejection, perhaps sensitise you to certain triggers, but not cause it. If you accept that you are born a manic depressive, then you can only learn how to live with it, adapt to it, survive it and live well.

Author's note

Like many people, John is unequivocal in his view that bipolar disorder is a psychoneurological illness. Central to this view is the theory of neurological susceptibility to a transmission dysfunction at the synaptic junction, leading episodically to the disinhibition and excitement of manic flights and the apathy and despair of depressive troughs. It is a susceptibility that can be reduced by the use of mood stabilising drugs such as lithium.

John's story, while at variance with the philosophical thrust of this book, represents a widely held view of bipolar disorder, a view taken by many of my colleagues in the psychiatric professions and by many people using mental health services who are subject to wildly fluctuating moods.

I would simply ask whether we can ever completely disentangle our moods from the flow of life events that impinged on our consciousness and are resonant in our unconscious? Is it helpful to see profound mood changes primarily as a neurological event? Of course, every action, every thought, every feeling, every perception has a neurophysiological basis, yet to understand the panoply of human behaviour simply in those terms is reductionism in the extreme. Is it not more human to take William Blake's view that

> *joy and woe are woven fine*
> *a clothing for the soul divine.*

My contention is that these polar opposites are present in us all, but for some the passions flow more freely in response to the cavalcade of life – an endowment that is both a blessing and a curse. Avoiding Olympian highs and Hadesian depths requires a person to walk prudently through life resisting the seductive call of both and yet still be able to retain a zest for living. I see John as someone who has been able to do this, in the process finding purpose and meaning in his work and family life which has helped anchor him in a life of reason and moderation.

The family dimension of recovery

4

*No man is an island
entire of itself.*

John Donne

Introduction

We live out our lives as part of many systems which both influence us and on which, in return, we have an influence. Among these, the family system is perhaps the most crucial to our psychological survival and wellbeing. It is therefore perverse that contemporary psychiatry continues to focus so much of its resources on the individual, locating problems within the referred patient, and conceptualising those problems as primarily biomedical or psychodynamic. Despite this there has been a growing recognition of the contribution that families make to the quality of life and to the return to wellbeing of someone who experiences a serious breakdown in their mental health. Of course, although less frequently referred to, the obverse is also true.

The needs of families are rightly high on the agenda of service priorities (Department of Health 1999, 2002b). Although family-orientated services have been slow to develop in Britain, there are examples of excellence. Since 1998 the Meriden West Midland Family Programme has trained over 2000 professionals of all disciplines in family work, through a system of cascade training. Suffolk Carers provides individual and group support, education and advocacy to families and offers training to carers and service users to enable them to participate more fully in the development of services.

There are over 600 000 people in Britain with enduring mental health problems. About 60% of them either live with their families or have frequent contact with them. It is of some significance then that studies of the family life of people who have experienced a serious breakdown in their mental health have, since the 1970s, consistently identified *high expressed emotion* as a reliable predictor of the course of such troubled states of mind (Bebbington & Kuipers 1994; Butzlaff & Hooley 1999). The key components of high expressed emotion in this context are: frequently expressed critical comments and hostility, reflecting feelings of frustration and anger experienced by relatives; and over-involvement which is driven by the guilt or anxiety felt by relatives. Neither reaction is conducive to recovery. In the first scenario a person is likely to experience a continuing state of tension and conflict, may feel rejected and become distant or dislocated from their family. In the second scenario increasing dependence and a loss of autonomy and confidence are likely to be the outcome. The use of the term *high expressed emotion* might seem to suggest that emotional neutrality is the social environment most conducive to recovery. That this is not so is reflected in the improved outcome for people who are sustained by the continuing, undemanding love of their families (Kuipers et al 2002).

Although the majority of people who experience enduring mental health problems live with their families, many others live in supported accommodation, or independent housing supported by community teams. The concept of high expressed emotion may be as relevant to staff teams and their interactions with their clients as it is to families (Tattan & Tarrier 2000).

This chapter considers in more detail the impact on the families of those suffering enduring mental health problems and the way these families might respond in a pragmatic and loving way to the challenges they face. The recovery journey can be liberating both for individual clients and for their families. It can be a process of learning and growth in which old attitudes and interactional patterns change and the family system becomes a more healing and sustaining system for everyone.

* * * * * * * * * * *

The family work approach most widely practiced within mental health services in Britain is behavioural family therapy. This is essentially a psycho-educational approach based on substantial research over the past 30 years into the role of negative *high expressed emotions* in perpetuating distressed, disturbed and dysfunctional behaviour. While the research data supporting its efficacy are impressive, it has been criticised for being too formulaic in its interventions and too dogmatic in its endorsement of the view that vulnerability to psychosis is biologically determined (Aderhold & Gottwalz 2004; Read et al 2004). It is argued that it sidesteps the role of dysfunctional elements in family life as one of many factors determining vulnerability, as was proposed when the vulnerability–stress model of psychosis was first conceived (Zubin & Spring 1977). In doing so, it seals off the possibility of a more open discussion of family dynamics and the opportunity for a more profound therapeutic journey for all the family.

Families, guilt and blame

Since the 1960s, when R.D. Laing thrust the idea of pathogenic families into public awareness, there has been an anxiety around apportioning blame. This notion of family culpability is bitingly illustrated in Philip Larkin's poem 'This be the Verse', which begins 'They fuck you up, your mum and dad / they may not mean to but they do', before continuing more redeemingly, if pessimistically, 'but they were fucked up in their turn / by fools in old-style coats and hats'. Clearly there is no desire on the part of mental health professionals to alienate families, most of whom are deeply caring and feel great sadness, anguish, bewilderment and remorse at the suffering of their children. But avoiding this issue can lead to a collusive engagement that attributes all dysfunction to processes within the diagnosed individual. This may assuage some parental guilt, but in my experience many families, perhaps most, simply do not believe it. Even after participating in psycho-educational family work which promulgates a biologically based vulnerability–stress model of psychosis, guilt and remorse not only remain but can be accentuated. What is not talked about grows in significance in the minds of relatives.

It is deeply distressing to feel that in some way you may have been responsible for the troubled state of mind of someone you love, but mitigation and peace of mind come not from avoiding these issues but from confronting them. In the light of open, sometimes painful exploration, families come to see that their parental fallibilities and the family discord they have presided over is not entirely of their choosing or design but emerges from the complex psychodynamics of family life, which are often intergenerational and transposed from their family of origin. Adverse socioeconomic factors too can exacerbate the tensions a family system tries to contain and which erupt in discordant relationships. None of this of course in any way absolves us as parents from responsibility for any neglect, hurt or abuse we may inflict on a child but it can free us from the punishing burden of guilt and open up the pathway to forgiveness and reconciliation.

The suicide of my eldest son on the cusp of the new millennium has caused me and my family an enormous amount of painful soul searching. The guilt was so engulfing that it felt for a while as if my life was no longer tenable. I could see nothing for me in a life that included such a painful reality. All joy was extinguished, all meaning shattered. I felt that all my faults and fallibilities, as a man, as a father, as someone who has made his career in psychiatric care, had been exposed, despite the loving support of many people, who urged me not to blame myself.

My son was one of twin boys whose brother died in infancy. We were not good as a family at honouring the short life of his dead twin, either in family conversations or memorialising rituals: memories of that devastating event were too raw, and as a result my son grew up with only a sketchy knowledge of his twin and the circumstances of his death. In one of our rare conversations about his brother's death I recall him saying – the poignancy of that moment still achingly fresh in my mind – 'It must have been difficult for you to love me after he died'. I now believe that, despite being only three months old at the time of his twin's death, he carried some survivor guilt into adult life. Of course he was cherished and loved completely, but what mattered was his perception, and loud and clear in that question from the heart was a huge amount of doubt.

Given to moods of melancholy throughout my life I know that I was at times a brooding and morose presence in my family. My father was of a similar nature and I recall how, caught in those saturnine moods, he often seemed unloving and disapproving. There was little emotional discourse and family frictions and feuds usually continued unresolved until nullified by some interceding event. So much of life in my family of origin seemed to centre on pleasing, or at least not upsetting, my father. I grew up a quiet, fearful, emotionally illiterate child with little inner sense of self-worth. Part of this emotional landscape was, I now recognise, recreated in my own family as my children were growing up. Feelings were not a welcome currency of communication and we all knew more about containing feelings than expressing them. Such an emotionally muted upbringing may have deprived my son of the emotional education necessary to deal with the tempests that blow through every life.

Ben Okri, in his book *The Famished Road*, talks about the 'spirit children': children who have no wish to be born, who do not feel at home in this life and are only anchored here by love. Though my twin boys were deeply loved it was somehow not fierce enough to hold them here. Despite being a talented artist, who was regarded with affection and appreciation by many people, it was in the end not enough to sustain his sense of self-worth, not enough to convince him of the value of his life, in the face of the phantoms of persecution that had gathered about him.

Families as a source of mental health

I have come to believe that the pre-eminent function of family life is to provide a loving cup. Parental care which is emotionally nurturing provides us with a protective inoculation against the adversities and misfortunes of life, a resilience boosted by subsequent advantageous life events. In one of the most influential studies of the emotional life of families over the past 50 years, John Bowlby underlined the significance of secure attachment between parent and child in conferring emotional resilience and a propensity to good mental health (Bowlby 1988). Attachment is not of course something that ends with childhood but is a bond we seek to replicate throughout life in our most intimate adult relationships. We break and remake many affectional bonds in the course of our lives, bonds which sustain us to a greater or lesser degree, often revealing the same patterns of secure or insecure attachment behaviour that existed in the parental relationship (Ainsworth 1991). Our family and marital attachment relationships, even loving friendships, provide us with that all-important secure base from which to engage fully in life, to explore our destinies and to grow.

For the process of recovery to move forward, clients need that safe base. An important focus of family work is for the therapist to enter the family system and facilitate an interaction which enables the family to provide that crucial emotionally supportive function. Where a family or social support network is absent or inaccessible, mental health professionals or the care team may be alone in providing that safe base from which a client begins the recovery journey. Secure attachment relationships with mental health professionals, if sustained, allow a process of internalisation to take place so that even when the attachment figure is not available the internalised 'good object' provides a source of confidence and supports autonomous behaviour (Byng-Hall 1995). This factor can be neglected in planning recovery services where long-term relationships, staff availability and expanded contact time could be key aspects of therapeutic effectiveness. Of course there will always be staff changes but if the team has a collaborative responsibility for a client, the safe base remains intact even though a key worker might leave.

Relationship realignment

One of most difficult aspects of recovery for families is in the area of what we might call relationship realignment. The enduring nature of some mental health problems, particularly those that emerge in adolescence and early adulthood, disrupts normal developmental changes within a family system. As we move towards adult maturity it is usual for there to be a gradual loosening of attachments to allow some separation to take place, autonomy and independence to grow and new attachment relationships to be formed. The onset of a lengthy period of distress and dysfunction, whether manifested in disabling anxiety, engulfing depression or a disturbing break with consensual reality, can lead to a regressive realignment within the family system.

This scenario can be played out in many ways. The increasing dependency of a young adult may for a while be accepted by one or both parents. This increased parental care and supervision may be acceded to and can be necessary for a time, but the negative corollary is that it can shade into parental over-involvement and lead to helplessness and loss of confidence. Alternatively it may provoke angry resentment – the young person, despite the disabling or distressing nature of their experience, wants to taste the same freedom, responsibility and autonomy as their peers. Another variation of this scenario is that one or both parents may critically reject the increasing dependency needs of their son or daughter, with resultant discord within the family, sometimes leading to splitting, distancing or separation. Similarly the sibling bond may be weakened by growing resentment about the demands a brother or sister is making on the emotional resources of the family. It is easy to see how the manifestation of distress in an individual can disrupt the balance and alignment of relationships within the family and undermine the system as a safe base from which family members can continue to grow and function confidently in the world.

Sometimes realigned relationships become very entangled and dysfunctional. In one family I know the mother became enmeshed with her teenage daughter who for a time had been adrift in a floridly psychotic world. Although living separately, her mother continued to do most things for her, in the process excluding the input of her support worker. This enmeshment arose partly out of maternal guilt and protectiveness, but also filled an emptiness in the mother's own life. The mother's relationship with her other daughters was weakened as a consequence of this over-involvement, as was the daughter's relationship with her siblings.

In another family I encountered, the daughter, who has a long history of para-noid anxiety, split her parents and assumed the authority of the parental subsystem, running the home like an open prison in which she was the often oppressive senior warder. In doing so she was attempting to manage her over-whelming anxieties by regulating contact between the outside world and the home and maintaining close proximity to her parents.

The configuration of the family system in dysfunctional ways may be more than a reaction to the onset of distress behaviour. It may be an exacerbation of attachment patterns which have existed for a long time and which have contributed to an individual's growing distress. An example of this is a family whose son had been referred to mental health services with an increasingly dis-abling thought disorder. The parents, Don and Jude, had two children: Euwan, the referred client, and Rebecca, the eldest child, who worked away from home. Euwan had become ensnared in ruminative thoughts about esoteric cosmo-logical and astrological ideas. Accompanying this was a pervasive uncertainty which caused him to prevaricate about everything. Making decisions was a tortuous process which at times immobilised him. This created considerable anxiety for his parents who needed to resume a caretaking presence in his life. Problems began to arise because of Don's growing over-involvement in his son's life, motivated by high levels of anxiety and guilt. This led to a weakening of the parents' bond with each other and they became more distant as a couple, disagreeing vehemently about the best way to respond to Euwan's behaviour. Though essentially loving and respectful towards his parents, Euwan was highly ambivalent about their increased involvement in his life. At times he could be acquiescent and at other times rejecting; a similar ambivalence existed towards the mental health services. Although he was troubled and lost in a psychological maze, he seemed determined to find his own way out.

At a time when the parents needed to be a strong unit, working together to provide consistent and coherent care, they were being pulled apart. It became clear that both were becoming stressed to breaking point and that their own mental health was beginning to suffer. They began to experience a sense of despondency about the prospect of Euwan's recovery, seeing their role as carers stretching unendingly on into the future. In this was a great deal of sadness that the opportunities in life that Euwan was on the threshold of being able to seize were slipping away unlived. There was also remorse that they had been neg-ligent in not putting a stop to Euwan's experimentation with cannabis which they believed was a significant causative factor.

Although the parents were reticent about their own families of origin, we sensed that they had both experienced difficult upbringings. Both had to grow up quickly and become self-reliant emotionally. Jude adopted the mask of a tough minded woman and Don that of a self-contained man. Although there was undoubtedly 'a kind of loving' between them it seemed hard for them to communicate and respond to each other's emotional needs.

Why is it that so many young men experience a breakdown in their mental health in the transition to adulthood? Traditionally the transitional journey to young adulthood for males is presided over by men. It is in the society of men that adolescents learn what masculinity means and how to channel their adult desires and aspirations. Harrop & Trower (2001) have commented on how the tasks of adolescence can often provoke similar traits to those often seen in psychosis: marked shifts in mood and self-esteem, self-consciousness, grandiosity; fluctuations between uncertainty and certitude and an indulgence in fantastical lives. Much of this was apparent in Euwan's behaviour. Coming through this testing passage requires the presence of parental figures who continue to provide emotional and mental grounding so that these young men do not, like Icarus in his flight of freedom, fly too close to the sun.

Virginia Satir, one of the pioneers of family therapy, wisely observed: 'All of the ingredients of family life that count, are changeable and correctable – individual self worth, communication, the system, the rules, at any point in time' (Satir 1972). A change has occurred in this family: there has been a realignment of relationships. Euwan and his father are not so enmeshed and a closer adult–adult relationship seems to be emerging. Don has been able to manage his anxieties about Euwan sufficiently to allow him the freedom to find his way. The parents' relationship is stronger and they have been able to lay claim to a life for themselves both as a couple and as individuals. Overall the sum of positive emotional energy in the family has increased. We developed a real affection and regard for the family during our work with them. They showed great resolve while this storm was blowing through their lives and demonstrated unstinting love towards Euwan, ensuring that his social moorings to family and friends were not dislocated as he struggled to find his road to recovery.

As we see in the above scenario, when a family member experiences a serious breakdown in their mental health there can be significant feelings of loss akin to a grief reaction, particularly if that breakdown persists. There may be some denial of the seriousness of the problem, perhaps seeing dysfunctional behaviour as a developmental phase or as a neurotic episode that will pass. As the distress behaviour continues, denial gives way to angry protest which may be self-directed, expressing itself in punishing blame and guilt. It may be directed at the troubled individual who is angrily accused of being lazy, of not trying hard enough to overcome their difficulties, of being selfish and self-centred or of being a fantasist. Often mental health professionals become the target of the family's protest at the unjustness of what has happened and are castigated for failing to provide effective treatment or adequate care. There may be a desperate search for an answer or for signs that the disorder is improving. Beyond this there are feelings of sadness and despair as a loved one's dysfunctional state of mind continues, associated with the pain of witnessing the troubled, chaotic world they now inhabit. There may be grieving for a lost emotional connection; for the person they used to be; and for lost dreams and aspirations. As time moves on there can be lingering grief about the loss of one's own life in the process of caring.

Eventually grief gives way to a state of acceptance, an attitude of mind which is more than mere resignation. Resignation is a capitulation, a giving up and passively allowing events of a seemingly overwhelming nature to run their course. Acceptance is different. It means that we are able to acknowledge the reality of the situation and live with that reality without losing our emotional equilibrium. We are not oppressed or depressed by it but are able to integrate it into an essentially positive view of life. From this position it is possible to see beyond vulnerabilities, to see again a person's worth, to see their qualities and strengths, to see the possibilities and opportunities in a life that has changed. It is at this point that families can become a positive force in a loved one's recovery journey.

Support for carers and families

Once a person's troubled state of mind and the accompanying distress has been diagnosed, dysfunction is designated 'sick role' behaviour and for a time is legitimised. The overriding feeling is one of sympathy and concern and unusual or antisocial behaviour, provided it is not too extreme, is tolerated by the family and neighbourhood. But there comes a point where frustration at an unchanging situation in which the family is exposed to ongoing difficult behaviour causes compassion fatigue to set in. Then care and concern turn to criticism and resentment. As one parent said to me after many years of giving loving, unfailing support to her son through recurrent periods of turbulence, 'I feel guilty saying this but there are times when I wish he was dead.'

Relatives may have to cope with an array of unusual and difficult behaviour, often on a daily basis. There may be withdrawn, asocial behaviour; abuse and aggression; separation anxiety demanding the continuing presence of a parent or spouse; lethargy and apathy; emotional indifference; delusional preoccupations; obsessional ruminations; hallucinatory responses; and potentially unsafe behaviour. Living with asocial, bewildering, inaccessible, unaesthetic, threatening, chaotic or unsafe behaviour can seriously deplete a family's emotional resilience and come to dominate their lives. One carer describes how living with someone who at the time was unable or unwilling to recover his own life left her with a desperate need to recover her own (in Massey et al 2005):

> The chaos that ensues is emotional, physical, practical and social. It threatens the ability to love and cherish. It prompts a desire to get away. It engenders denial and a need to be absolved of guilt. Sometimes it gives rise to real fear for the personal safety of everyone involved. Jobs are threatened and friendships seriously disrupted. This is a personal disaster which rips apart the fabric of life, challenging values and distressingly altering expectations for the future.

There is a need for a collaborative partnership between clients, their families and mental health professionals and this can be enhanced through sharing information. A diagnosis of schizophrenia or bipolar disorder requires explanation as does the aetiology, symptomatology, treatment and likely outcome. This increased understanding of dysfunctional behaviour can be helpful in modifying attitudes and influencing family interaction. While a medical interpretation of dysfunctional behaviour may be valued by some families, I have found that a discussion of the stress–vulnerability model, which sees both a person's vulnerability and their distress as arising out of their lived experience, a much more acceptable approach. From this point of departure the client, the family and mental health professional can embark on a journey of discovery, which will eventually lead in the direction of recovery. So, for example, psychosocial withdrawal, 'duvet diving' and hearing critical voices may be primarily associated with someone's social anxiety and low self-esteem, which has arisen out of their experience of insecure attachments, the loss of a safe base and being systematically bullied at school. This kind of insight opens up a pathway to recovery through developing secure attachments, building self-esteem, supported social re-engagement and trauma counselling.

The majority of complaints and criticism that families have about their relatives are related to so-called negative symptoms: apathy, inertia, withdrawal, dysfunctional thoughts and inverted sleep patterns (Kuipers et al 2002). Usually creative solutions are possible. Narrative therapy is one approach that has been used effectively with clients who have a previous diagnosis of schizophrenia and is a valuable strategy for supporting the resolve and creativity of families in overcoming the difficulties they encounter with the family member's behaviour (White & Epston 1990). By externalising the problem, conflict that has built up around it decreases and the client and family are united in a collaborative effort to free their lives and relationships from its influence. This approach results in the problem becoming differentiated from the person. The problem then becomes the problem, not the person!

Externalising is a function of the questioning; Since this *shut down living* has had a grip on your lives, what effect does it have on you individually and on your relationships?' 'Since '*the voices*' have been around how have they interfered with family life?' I find it useful to encourage families to define the problem in their own way rather than use the language of psychiatry. This frees the complained of behaviour from pathology, normalises it and encourages a more active problem resolution stance. Interestingly it is common for the process of externalisation to prompt a revision of the family narrative. Creating some space in the family's story that has been so dominated by the problem allows more positive elements of their lives and relationships to emerge in an emotionally sustaining form.

Once the problem has been externalised and elaborated, the family is encouraged to map its influence on the problem. There may be occasions in the past when the client and/or the family have had the upper hand over the problem; times when they reacted differently, in a way that made a difference, resulting in a *unique outcome.* Sometimes it can be difficult for families to identify any occasions in which they have had such an influence, particularly if they are feeling powerless in the face of a longstanding, seemingly intractable problem. But usually, having revealed their influence over the problem, they are less transfixed by it and are galvanised into identifying their competence and resourcefulness in the face of this adversity.

Sometimes problem behaviour can be improved by limit setting. The complained of behaviour may continue precisely because there has not been clear communication between family members about what is acceptable. Sometimes limits have been set but might have been imposed in a hostile, critical way, as a result provoking some resistance. Limit setting should be a reciprocal activity, with the client benefiting from being supported in asserting his/her right to make an autonomous decision. So, for example, in the case of one client I know, his autonomous choice is to live in a state of spartan orderliness which is contrary to his family's assessment of what constitutes minimal comfort.

If recovery is to be encouraged there needs to be some element of risk-taking, regardless of fears about the wellbeing of a loved one, if they are to be allowed more independence: fears about exploitation, assault, self-harm or suicide; fears about a neglect of self-care or social exclusion and isolation; fears about a worsening of their mental health. It is important to check out the validity of the concerns. Often the fears have more to do with exaggerated parental anxieties than with social realities, but they can severely restrict everyone's lifestyle. If we stayed within the boundaries of what was safe and known, little personal development would ever take place. We must be prepared to take the risk of allowing people their independence, their freedom to try. To use Samuel Beckett's phrase 'To try and fail. No matter. Try again, fail better'.

Being a carer can be stressful. Even where a relative is living independently or in supported housing, it can be difficult to let go of the burden of care and concern sufficiently to have enough energy free for a life of one's own. The stressors that have already been identified in this chapter can be unremitting and hard to bear unsupported. The government has a commitment to increase by 700 the number of carer support workers active within the mental health field (Department of Health 2000). Such a commitment has yet to be fully realised and one must conclude that many families are continuing to struggle on, largely unsupported. Carers need emotional support, information and practical advice and periodic respite from caring. Many can benefit from the kind of family work outlined in this chapter. Current guidelines recommend that family interventions should take place over at least six months and involve a minimum of ten sessions (National Institute for Health and Clinical Excellence 2002).

There is often a legacy of disaffection with mental health services. Families may have come over time to feel disregarded by professionals, uninformed and uninvolved. They are left feeling that their knowledge of their kith and kin and the care they provide are unimportant. Or that they are blamed for their relative's misfortune. Or they may perhaps have been labelled as 'fusspots' or 'complainers' by staff who may only have had contact with them during crisis episodes, when emotions are likely to have been highly charged. Working through these misperceptions and their associated negativity is a necessary starting point in building a collaborative relationship with carers for support workers or family therapists, particularly if those workers are linked directly with mental health services.

Finally, it would be a mistake to think that all family caring is a harrowing experience. I have met many families who have enjoyed new dimensions to their relationship with a loved one, whose life course and way of being in the world has been inextricably altered by their psychological turmoil. Previous aspirations and expectations may have dissolved like dreams, but waking to the new dawn offers fresh possibilities and opportunities for a life of value and fulfilment. If families accept this proposition they can act as guardians of hope and find joy in the emergence of this new life as recovery proceeds. The case for the therapeutic support of families is overwhelming as an element in recovery. Through sharing the recovery journey they can find a way of being as a family and as individuals that is more emotionally sustaining and life enhancing than that which may have existed before the family member's breakdown. In this sense recovery can be truly a family experience

To hell and back – a personal reflection on recovery

Emma

My relationship with the mental health services has been a long one. I had a pretty dysfunctional childhood although I do retain some good memories of my very early life. At the age of seven my behaviour changed markedly as I became very 'accident-prone' repeatedly 'falling' down stairs and having other 'accidents'.

I recall hoping to become injured so I could escape the home situation without doing what I had been forbidden to do, which was to tell anyone what was happening when my mother was at work. It didn't work and my torment continued. In time my family grew and I had three brothers. The abuse and accompanying threats continued and escalated; it would be all my fault, the boys would go into care and hate me and my mum wouldn't believe me or love me. So I said nothing.

At the age of eleven, after a particularly bad weekend, I went to school knowing that I could no longer deal with life. I believed that if I were no longer on the planet then my torment would be over and my family and my mum would be saved somehow. I hung myself in the gym changing room from the overhead pipes with a makeshift noose. Another pupil came in, raised the alarm and I was cut down, unconscious with severe bruising to my throat.

So began my involvement with services. I was made to see an educational psychologist but I hated it. She came to school and I was pulled out of lessons to see her. Other pupils started asking me who I was seeing and why, but I had no answers. It made me different. I was often teased and bullied, 'the nutter seeing a shrink'. I decided that I would have to bury my feelings in order to survive and get out of seeing this woman. In what was to be our last session I told her that I hated her and wanted her dead. She never came back.

I changed schools due to a family move shortly after, but my plan to ignore feelings was failing and I began to cut myself to feel like I had some degree of control within the chaos of my life. When I was thirteen I overdosed on paracetamol. Looking back I don't know whether I specifically wanted to be dead or simply wanted out of my situation. Much to my horror I ended up in an adolescent psychiatric unit. It felt like leaving the frying pan for the safety of the fire. I was scared, alone and untrusting. I begged to go home – at least that was familiar. After two weeks I got my wish.

My self-harm continued as I battled to cope with life and growing up. At 15 I was held by the police for my own safety and was placed on an adult ward of the local psychiatric hospital on a section, as there were no adolescent beds available. The staff were unapproachable, other patients felt threatening, medication was insisted on but not explained. I felt more violated than ever. After three days I was moved to the adolescent unit. It felt like a prison, privileges had to be earned, punishments for non-compliance included being 'put in pyjamas' where all your possessions were removed until the staff deemed you worthy of their return. After eight months all it did for me was to confirm my opinion that I was worthless and must have done something very bad for people to behave in the way they were.

I continued life seeing various professionals periodically. The most memorable session was with a psychologist who, in an attempt to show me just how 'lucky' I was, took me to the bedside of a young teenage boy in the children's ward. He had been hit by a car and was looking at a life of severe physical and mental impairment.

As I looked at him I remember thinking how I wished it were me in the bed. So much for improving my self-worth!

At the age of 18 I was being treated for the effects of yet another overdose in the general hospital when I looked in my notes only to find, right at the front, scrawled on a square yellow post-it note 'personality disordered?' So now I had a reason for how I was and surely that would mean that if the doctors knew what was wrong they could fix it. I was so relieved – but so wrong. Nobody would talk to me to explain how the diagnosis was reached, what help was available or even whether I could ever feel better than I had for so long already in my short life.

My existence continued into my twenties, doing a degree, working part-time, self-harming and searching for peace within myself. It seemed so easy for others to progress, develop and grow while I spent endless hours pursuing destructive relationships in my quest to feel normal.

By 24 I felt that I had lost the battle with my demons. In desperation to bring a final conclusion to my situation I had dared to ask for help from the people whom I distrusted most, the doctors. They had given my condition a name but then used that to tell me that there was no treatment, no hope of improvement or change. I had no future. I left the doctors' office and knew that I had reached the end. I climbed on the roof of the hospital but was stopped from jumping by a male nurse who had seen me and followed.

And so I found myself on a section being held on a locked ward. I initially felt relief, as now they, the doctors, would have to do something to help. In reality it meant that I found myself in an even more emotionally charged position where my first attempt to harm myself led to four months of being 'specialled'. I have to say I didn't feel very special! I'm sure that if you put anyone in a situation where they are watched at arm's length 24/7, most would crack. I couldn't even have a crap in peace. I would wake in the night as staff at my bedside sat chatting to each other. It was far from therapeutic, and I still managed to self-harm, so what did it achieve other than create a 'them and us' attitude and lower my self-image even further than I believed possible?

With the help of friends that I had met in a self-help group I found out about a unit in London specifically for self-harmers and repeatedly asked to be referred. Eventually my consultant reluctantly agreed if only to wash his hands of me. That was my turning point. I was assessed and accepted for a six month programme of treatment. For the first time in years I felt that I not only had some control of my situation but I had hope. The programme was intense and hard, numerous therapy groups, one on one sessions and activity nights, but also endless support and encouragement from both staff and other residents. I had to take responsibility for my actions; I was allowed choice in my self-harming. That was important as it negated the need to hide what I was doing to myself. When I felt the need to harm I could speak to staff about how I was feeling, possible triggers and most importantly alternatives to harming.

When I left the unit I returned to the care of my local hospital and was allocated a community psychiatric nurse. She continued to support me and tried to understand me and in return I slowly continued in my recovery. She often said that I would see light at the end of the tunnel. I would tell her that the tunnel I was in had loads of twists and turns so I couldn't always see it. She stayed with me through everything and even defended me when doctors were less than understanding. One time I took a large valium overdose but was found collapsed. When I told the junior doctor shortly afterwards during an admission assessment he told me bluntly that if I had taken as many as I said then I would be dead. My CPN was present and confirmed what I had told him and admonished him immediately. I knew I had an ally.

Although there were still many mountains to climb, I developed a new attitude towards life. I knew I ultimately held the key to my own recovery so I adopted a 'shit happens' mantra. Whatever was thrown at me would be something to deal with before moving on. My CPN eventually moved on but told me well in advance so that we could work through the feelings of abandonment that had accompanied every other ending of relationship that I had experienced. She introduced me to a new worker and we had joint meetings so that the trauma I felt was minimal. I felt that I had a part in the decisions made in my care – nothing was dictated. This helped me to feel in control to the point that I rarely hurt myself.

I had a new consultant who realised the need for two-way communication in my care. I have continued on my journey to wellness. I have many regrets regarding my time spent with the services: the fact that I have spent the best part of my teens and twenties just existing; that much of my time in the services felt like worse abuse than I initially faced at home; that problems weren't dealt with effectively in the first place before escalating to the point that they did.

However, I now don't regret having to make my journey as it has shaped me into the person I am today. And of that I am proud. I am working with professionals to try to ensure that the people who enter the system in the future get a far higher standard of care and effective early treatment so that in years to come people do not have to endure the sort of negative experience that I endured for so long.

I am a member of a group born out of the clinical governance process, looking at effective interventions for people deemed to have personality disorder. This group comprises psychiatrists, nurses, social workers and other interested parties, including me. We have held a conference at which I ran a workshop on self-help. It generated a great deal of interest and enthusiasm, with most professionals recognising the considerable need for improvement. However, several years down the line and after an initial show of interest from those holding the purse strings, there is now no money available to develop the project further. While I understand the dire state of NHS finances, I remain incredulous about the wisdom of the short-term view being taken. In my book it makes more sense to spend a relatively small amount on early, effective intervention if such action results in huge financial savings from avoided inpatient care, not to mention reducing the emotional cost to individuals, their families and society as a whole.

I was told many times that there was no point in trying to help me as I would always be this way until I killed myself. I would like to tell all those doubters that that is not my fate any more. I have not hurt myself for more than five years. I met a wonderful man and have been married for nearly a year, and I have obtained and retained a full time job for over a year. I am now a worthwhile and contributing member of society, which is all I really wanted to begin with.

The cultural and community dimension of recovery

5

Our predicament is the world – the social environment – in which we live; our suffering arises from our relations with it.

David Smail

Introduction

There is an important social dimension to recovery. People who have a history of disabling distress often find themselves marginalised, oppressed and stigmatised by society. Not only do they have to cope with a vulnerability to severe and disabling psychological distress but also with humiliating discrimination, which results in them becoming among the most excluded in society (Sayce 2000). Being part of the social fabric of the community is necessary for our psychological survival. Unemployment, poverty, poor housing or homelessness and social isolation – common experiences among people with enduring mental health problems – are not a recipe for sustained wellbeing. The better outcomes for people with severe mental health problems in developing countries when compared with industrialised nations point to the preservation of social connections and employment opportunities as key factors in promoting recovery and sustaining mental health (Jablensky et al 1992).

Social inclusion and full citizenship can have a greater positive impact on recovery than any other factor and should therefore be at the top of the agenda for mental health workers seeking to work in a recovery-orientated way. Yet as mental health professionals we often become overly focused on the inner life of the individual, believing that if we can help heal the psyche then the social dimension of a person's life will improve. In doing so we are ignoring the lessons of history that provide ample evidence that the greatest gains in health and wellbeing have come from initiatives that improve conditions of living. It seems to me that often more can be gained by standing alongside people in their struggle to overcome social adversity and injustice than through psychotherapeutic or pharmacological interventions.

Social exclusion is not just a barrier to recovery but compounds the mental health problems people face. Studies of institutional life over three decades ago highlighted the profoundly damaging effects on identity and autonomy of impoverishing, disempowering, institutional regimes (Wing 1970; Barton 1976). Thankfully the wreckage of so many human lives is not seen today on the same scale; nevertheless the social experience of many people who enter the psychiatric system is still one of being marginalised and dehumanised. Recovering from the trauma, stigma and discrimination of becoming a psychiatric patient can be as difficult as recovering from the initial psychological disorder. Deegan (1997) argues, with good reason, that recovery is a politicised process that of necessity challenges the injustice that exists in the mental health care system and society at large.

I worked recently with a man who has come through fifteen years of being adrift in a psychotic world, five of which have been spent in a psychiatric hospital. He is now desperate to be allowed to 'grow up', to take charge of his own life. Every contact with services and with his family seems to reinforce a feeling of dependency and vulnerability. He lives in fear that every stray psychotic thought that percolates into his consciousness will betray him and lead to psychiatric services strengthening their grip on his life. For him, being discharged from services would equate with recovery because his unusual thoughts, perceptions and reclusive lifestyle would become just that – unusual rather than schizophrenic. His wish is to merge anonymously into the broad stream of life and seek to reinvent himself there, rather than to be diverted into a backwater of mental health resource centres and supported housing. He manages the fundamentals of day-to-day living well enough, but lives a solitary, unstructured existence and faces a tough challenge to find social acceptance and a life that has some measure of meaning and satisfaction. He is in fact facing a developmental task – the quest for identity, independence and autonomy, a task that most of us face in adolescence and early adulthood. It is a struggle that many people face in their recovery journey, to shed the cocoon of psychiatric care so that they may emerge reborn, transmuted from 'patient' to 'person', with the freedom and responsibility that is the right of all citizens. This is a man on the threshold of his recovery journey.

The barriers to social inclusion can seem insurmountable. It is sometimes easier to give up, to not care, to surrender to what Seligman (1975) described as learned helplessness. A psychiatric diagnosis and enduring mental health problems can seem to invalidate a person's right to exercise lifestyle choices and undermine efforts to realise personal aspirations. Such disempowerment and loss of control over one's life can be 'spirit breaking' and leads to apathy, withdrawal, resignation, submissiveness, depression, anxiety and anger – behaviour which is often interpreted as the negative symptoms of a psychotic disorder (Deegan 1992).

The chances of getting a job for someone who suffers a psychological breakdown are significantly reduced. A recent national survey revealed that up to 84% of people with a history of severe mental health problems were unemployed (Office of National Statistics 2000b) with an associated increase in poverty relative to their fellow citizens. In my own service, which supports 80 clients who have histories of persistent mental health problems, only 11% are working, or in full-time or part-time education, or engaged in significant voluntary work. Employers continue to discriminate against people with enduring mental health problems despite the evidence that employment success is not related to diagnosis or symptomatology (Repper & Perkins 2003). It has more to do with the availability of services and supports that rekindle the work ethic and the confidence needed to re-enter the employment arena.

Many people write themselves off as potential employees, having internalised the therapeutic pessimism of mental health professionals or having become over-identified with vulnerabilities and deficits so that confidence evaporates. Often there is a fear of failure and anxieties about exposing one's psychiatric past to employers and fellow workers. For others the burden of medication side-effects, or the disruptive nature of recurrent episodes of distress, make a return to work difficult. An additional disincentive to seek work is the complexity of the benefit system and the potential loss in income when moving from a benefit-based income to low paid employment. Yet a return to work remains, for many people, a benchmark in their recovery and opens the door to a more inclusive and rewarding lifestyle. The long recovery of John Nash, the Nobel Prize winning mathematician whose life was portrayed in the film *A Beautiful Mind*, from the paranoid world that engulfed his life took significant steps forward when he was enabled to return to Princeton University campus to resume his studies and eventually teach.

While there has been little recent research into the social causation of disabling psychological distress, there can be little doubt that the most impoverished people in society come off worse in any measure of health, either psychological or physical. What recent empirical evidence there has been confirms earlier findings that there is a correlation between low socioeconomic status, particularly in an urban context, and severe and enduring mental health problems (Marcelis et al 1998; Pedersen & Mortensen 2001). Living in deprived urban areas exposes people to more social stressors – poverty, pollution, noise, overcrowding, crime, violence, unemployment, drug misuse, social isolation. The primacy of social conditions rather than innate vulnerability as a causative factor in disabling psychological distress has been shamefully neglected and has often been obscured behind contentious notions such as the social drift theory that argues that people spiral down the socioeconomic order as a consequence of enduring psychological problems.

While countries like the UK which have enjoyed a relatively stable and growing economy make possible a more affluent lifestyle, this prosperity has not been distributed equitably. There is a growing underclass, a poorer section of the community who live on the margins of poverty, which includes a disproportionate number of people with persistent mental health problems. It is true that comparatively few people in Western society are homeless and hungry, yet not to be able to afford a lifestyle taken for granted by the majority leaves people feeling excluded.

Not only are poorer people exposed to more social stressors, they are also subject to a class bias in their contact with psychiatric services. They are more likely to be given a diagnosis of psychosis, more likely to be treated exclusively with drug regimens, more likely to be admitted compulsorily and spend longer in hospital than people higher up the socioeconomic order (Johnson 2000; Bindman et al 2002).

Friendships and social support networks tend to diminish in the wake of continuing mental health problems and family relationships may become distant or discordant. While the majority of people in Britain profess to have compassionate and inclusive attitudes towards those who experience a breakdown in their mental health (Ross & Read 2004), discrimination is still communicated in everyday social encounters in subtly distancing, patronising interactions, dismissive attitudes or overt hostility, leaving people feeling diminished and excluded from mainstream society. The stigmatising of psychiatric dis-ease remains a facet of community life, reinforced by tabloid portrayals of mental health sufferers involved in extreme incidents. Understandably people are often self-conscious about a psychiatric past, perhaps choosing to keep that aspect of their lives private, sometimes preferring to fabricate rather than speak openly about it. Others find it intolerable to have to live a life of deceit and opt to be disclosing in their social and occupational relationships. In doing so they boldly challenge the stigma that still exists in society and are ambassadors for all who struggle for acceptance.

Ethnicity and Mental Health

The difficulties faced by people in the social dimension of their lives are often compounded by issues related to race and gender. Despite a generation of multiculturalism and feminism, racism, misogyny and homophobia remain endemic in UK society. The tragic killing of Stephen Lawrence and Anthony Walker – both young men of considerable promise – is testimony to the deep roots of racism in society, and the death of David 'Rocky' Bennett in a psychiatric facility deepens the lingering shadow of institutional racism that hangs over psychiatric care. Such incidents can only have some redemptive meaning if they lead to the elimination from our society of racist attitudes at both a personal and an institutional level. The reality of racism within mental health services in Britain has been highlighted for the past 20 years by successive reports showing significant cultural variations in the experience of white British people and people from other ethnic groups (Box 5.1).

A young man with an Anglo-Caribbean background I have come to know over the past few years was arrested for stealing sandwiches from a supermarket and held in hospital on a section of the Mental Health Act for six months with a diagnosis of cannabis-induced psychosis. During his detention he was assessed as showing predominantly 'negative symptoms' of 'schizophrenia'. From his perspective, his symptoms were an expression of his feelings of disempowerment,

Box 5.1

Cultural variations in the experience of mental health services in Britain

Black people of Caribbean or African origin:

- Are more likely to be given a diagnosis of psychosis
- Are more likely to be admitted to a psychiatric hospital
- Are more likely to be detained under the Mental Health Act
- Are more likely to be referred through the courts or the police
- Are more likely to be placed in seclusion
- Are more likely to experience physical restraint
- Have higher levels of medication
- Spend longer in hospital
- Have less access to psychological therapies

(Adapted from the 'Count me in report' (Mental Health Act Commission 2005; Department of Health 2005))

the stultifying effects of medication and the emotional impact of the recent death of his father. I find it difficult to believe that this chapter in his life would have unfolded in this way had he been white British, assertively articulate and middle class.

Sadly, despite a raised consciousness of anti-discriminatory practice, we have to conclude that there is still a racist bias operating within mental health services. But that alone does not account for the statistical differences in diagnostic rates. It is the wider social experience of people from minority ethnic groups that accounts for this increased vulnerability. Any social group that encounters pernicious racist attitudes in everyday life, as well as higher levels of unemployment, poverty and social exclusion than the general population is bound to be at risk. A curious fact to emerge in recent research is that it is the children of first generation immigrant families who are particularly vulnerable (Bentall 2003). It is suggested that this may have something to do with schisms in cultural identity. People are faced with the difficult choice of integrating elements of both their culture of origin and the host culture into their identity, assimilating the host culture to the exclusion of the traditions and values of their cultural heritage, or separating from the host culture to maintain an identity rooted in their ethnicity. Ultimately individuals may end up marginalised by both the host culture and their culture of origin.

It is not hard to see how discrimination coupled with isolation and social disadvantage can play a significant role in the development of paranoid thinking and the manic episodes which form a common feature of the distress behaviour of people of Caribbean and African descent. A persecuted perspective on life will have some basis in fact and coping with the harsher realities of existence without despairing in a host culture that is not always benevolent gives rise to manic flights.

Table 5.1 Conditions for healing: a comparison of Eastern and Western traditions

Non-Western	Western
Harmony and balance	Problem solving
Acceptance	Control
Holistic understanding	Cognitive understanding
Harmony with social/spirit world	Body/mind/spirit separation
Unity of body-mind-spirit	Reintegration of the self
Traditional/alternative healers	Expert-led medical help
Experiential evidence	Empirically based medicine

This scenario is exemplified by a black British woman of my acquaintance with a long history of overwhelming distress typified by vacillating moods and troubled paranoid thoughts. She is the victim of a double jeopardy: that of being a black woman and a psychiatric patient in a society that discriminates against both. She identifies strongly with black culture, in which she has never found acceptance. Her dreams are of writing songs, of being a disc jockey, of finding 'her soul mate', yet she is so desolate and persecuted that often she can hardly bear to go out to the local shop. Because she does not feel at home in her identity she is caught in a web of doubt and uncertainty. Yet there are times when she laughs when her laughter seems to come from her soul. It comes bubbling up from the centre of her being and is earthy, joyful, strong, exuberant and warm and in those moments you know that this place will continue to call to her, urging her to begin her journey home.

The dominant discourse on severe distress is an ethnocentric Western view which, as we have seen in earlier chapters, conceptualises it as a dysfunctional state located within the individual. So dominant is this illness hypothesis that it has achieved the status of a truth and provides an authoritative basis for professional, expert-led care. While this conception may be relevant and acceptable to many, it is often inappropriate to people whose experience and beliefs are rooted outside Western cultures. The idea that recovery of wellbeing necessarily requires an intervention by mental health professionals is not a belief that is subscribed to by all cultures where ideas of what constitutes conditions for healing and recovery might have a different emphasis (Table 5.1). In many black African cultures traditional healers (diviners, herbalists, faith healers and shamans) are still consulted, sometimes along with doctors who are trained in Western medicine. Psychological distress is often understood as sorcery, as a manifestation of the displeasure of the ancestors, or as a reaction to social causes. Traditional healers use rituals, herbs, mojos, incantations and advice to harmonise the sufferer with their social and metaphysical worlds (Crawford & Lipsedge 2004).

But to think of culture as a fixed entity would be mistaken. It is an emergent process that is influenced by the social and family context as much as tradition (Fernando 1995). To make assumptions about people's mental health needs by reference to their ethnicity leads to stereotyping. Taking a more fluid view of culture frees us as mental health workers from relying too much on having a detailed knowledge of culture and faith traditions and allows us to draw much more on the specific experience of the individual and family in sensitively assessing needs. Cultural cross-pollination has undoubtedly taken place in the UK as non-Western philosophies and traditions relating to health and healing have permeated our multi-ethnic culture. The whole populace seems to have taken a step towards holistic and spiritual practices as an alternative to a passive reliance on scientific medicine.

Gender and mental health

There is persuasive evidence that differences exist in the social stressors to which men and women are exposed, leading to variations in the way mental health problems manifest themselves in women and in the way women experience mental health services. In its strategy document for the development of mental health care for women, the Department of Health (2002a) identify a number of socioeconomic and psychological factors that contribute to the higher incidence of mental ill health in women than in men. Women are more likely than men to be living in poverty. As primary carers for children, women face restricted employment opportunities, experience role overload and become socially isolated. They may be vulnerable to troubled states of mind and overwhelming distress following childbirth. They are more likely to suffer domestic violence and be victims of childhood sexual abuse.

In a review of 13 reputable studies Goodman et al (1997) estimated that between 51% and 97% of women experiencing psychosis reported being subjected to some form of abuse in their lifetime. In a further study of women with severe and persistent distress, Mueser et al (1998) found that 52% had been sexually abused during childhood. These are staggering figures, way above the average for the general population and strongly indicative of the role of trauma as a precursor or precipitant of severe psychological distress in adult life. Yet psychiatry offers little in the way of therapeutic attention to these traumatised women, many of whom show clear signs of post-traumatic stress disorder enmeshed with psychosis (Morrison et al 2003).

A woman I have been working with over the past few years who has a diagnosis of schizoaffective disorder bears many of the emotional scars of repeated trauma. She was abused physically in childhood and has been serially retraumatised by sexually exploitative and violent relationships in adult life. It is sometimes difficult to tell whether her accounts of sexual or physical assault are new or whether they are flashbacks to previous traumatic incidents. She finds the legacy of psychological pain hard to tolerate and copes by displacing it into an array of physical symptoms, misusing medication and comfort eating. Often she is despairing and experiences the world as a hostile and threatening place that at any moment is likely to deal her another blow. I sense that in the past the cause of her distress has not been fully heard or given sufficient credence in the clinical process of diagnosis and treatment. Yet she is a survivor who 'keeps on keeping on' despite the tides of emotional pain that flood her consciousness. It may seem an oversimplification, but her recovery is dependent on love. Over the years she has become accustomed to getting 'love' and 'care' in the form of pre-scribed drugs that make her feel better emotionally and physically. She regularly and desperately seeks changes in her prescription to cure the ache in her heart and soul. To be loved in an accepting undemanding way in the context of a per-sonal relationship, a family relationship, a friendship, or a therapeutic relation-ship would help heal the wounds caused by deprivation and abuse.

Many women continue to experience mental health service facilities as un-therapeutic partly because of the sexual harassment they encounter in mixed ward environments. In a study of 118 NHS trusts carried out by the Mental Health Act Commission, 56% reported problems relating to sexual harassment of women patients, ranging from assault to sexually disinhibited behaviour (Warner & Ford 1998). That a significant problem persists was confirmed by a study commissioned by Mind that found that one in six female patients had experienced sexual harassment (Baker 2000). Given that a substantial propor-tion of women have experienced sexual or physical abuse as children or adults, for that abuse to be replicated in hospital is an intolerable state of affairs. Clearly much work still has to be done to make services women friendly (if not women only), work which must go beyond issues of safety and privacy. Overall, as mental health workers we must develop a more sensitive understanding of the pressures in the lives of women that put them at greater risk of mental health problems.

It seems extraordinary that some 40 years after the philosophy of women's lib-eration began to permeate cultural consciousness we should still be addressing such fundamental issues in relation to women's mental health. How can we still be largely ignoring the traumas and social pressures that cause twice as many women as men to experience overwhelming psychological distress (Department of Health 2002a)? How is it that psychiatry is still dominated by male energies and agendas when more than ever we need a feminisation of mental health services, a transition that would promote a more compassionate, person-centred, contextualised approach to care that no longer sees patients as symp-tom entities. Perhaps the heart of the problem lies in wider society where elements of patriarchy and misogyny remain and reveal themselves in the con-tinuing inequality and oppression in the lives of many women. Although we might wish it to be otherwise, public services, stripped of any refinement, reflect the prevailing mores and ethics of the society they serve.

Overshadowed by the necessary debate about women's health, men's mental health issues are often neglected. But they are real and worrying. Young men seem particularly vulnerable to distressed troubled states of mind, reflected most strikingly in the higher suicide rates. A snapshot of the young men (under 35) on the case load of my own service, all of whom have a diagnosis of psychosis, reveals that 90% are unemployed and have not had significant work experience, 70% had absent or distant fathers during their formative years, 90% have no experience of a sustained personal or sexual relationship, 80% have no friend-ship network, 93% have been or are regular or heavy users of street drugs. Although this is a small sample statistically, it highlights the poverty of oppor-tunity for the kind of social learning experiences necessary for a transition to mature adulthood. What I notice often in these young men is an attitude that implies a 'resignation from life', as if their dreams and aspirations have shriv-elled on the vine and they have settled into an apathetic, sometimes angry, isol-ated existence. Viewed from such an alienated position it can be hard for them to see a positive future for themselves.

Tremendous change has taken place in the lives of men over the last 50 years. The declining industrial base and the disappearance of labour intensive indus-tries robbed men of the occupational roles from which they once drew their sense of identity. Young men are no longer exposed to the 'lessons in masculin-ity' that were once absorbed from the work culture. The 'new man' who began to emerge in the liberal culture of the 1960s which created a social climate in which men could develop their feminine side has left men feeling incomplete. While there is satisfaction for men in being able to develop and express their more caring, feeling side, it has been at the expense of their positive masculine energy, referred to by Robert Bly in his insightful book *Iron John* as the 'Inner Warrior' (Bly 1990). When energised, this male archetype strengthens and ennobles men with boldness, fortitude, competitiveness, vigour, honour and pride. There needs to be a balance. To be defined mainly by qualities normally associated with femininity can be threatening to most men and to be an unre-formed dominant male is no longer acceptable in a culture of equality. We have also seen male aggression and sexuality demonised in our culture, where they have become associated with domestic violence, child abuse and violent crime. This is an image which makes it difficult to accept and integrate positive mas-culine energy and allow it to infuse the personality and to be expressed in con-structive ways.

The 1960s also saw the emergence of a vibrant and vocal feminist movement which challenged inequalities between the sexes and the subordinate role of women in society. As a result of this cultural shift, women are no longer so dependent on men and men no longer the sole providers and protectors of the family. This and the high divorce rate continue to have a significant impact on the psychological and physical health of men. While many women seem to enjoy a greater sense of wellbeing in the wake of marital breakdown, men show an increase in mental and physical health problems, suggesting that while being in a long-term cohabiting relationship is good for men, it is less so for women.

Embedded in the Western psyche is the idea that women are more vulnerable and needy emotionally, more emotionally literate and socially adept. Men are per-ceived as more emotionally constrained or suppressed, needing less emotional sustenance from their relationships. It is of course a stereotype but one that has sufficient power to make it difficult for men to acknowledged their distress.

Men who have not found a place in society, who have no concept of what it is to be a man, are prey to a desperate sense of alienation and depression. This crisis of identity and self-esteem can be seen in the suicide rates, the early onset of severely troubled states of mind, the widespread use of street drugs and problem drinking. What is missing most from the lives of many young men is the presence of positive role models of masculinity. There is an urgent need for elders and mentors to assume this role. What it is to be a man can only be learned from other men, from their example and from their stories.

Facilitating social inclusion

So where does that leave us at the end of this reflection on the social dimension of recovery? It is of course easier to point out the barriers to recovery than it is to overcome them. But positive change is happening, albeit slowly. The majority of people in Britain do have a compassionate, inclusive attitude towards those who experience a breakdown in their mental health. Discriminatory practices within mental health services are being challenged and reformed. The proposed reform of the incapacity benefit does seem to reflect a genuine attempt on the part of government to help the long-term sick back into work, a proposal that is not simply aimed at reducing the cost to the nation of sickness benefit, but also demonstrates a concern for people's sense of worth and dignity. Innovative mental health resource centres exist which embrace people in an enabling, inspiring spirit of community, and provide a stepping stone to social integration. Imaginative Social Enterprise projects offer realistic work opportunities and a transitional pathway to unsupported employment. Supported housing projects provide a route to independent tenancies for people who have not been able to establish or maintain a home of their own.

And yet for many people who have experienced severe and disabling distress, social inclusion and full citizenship still seems a faraway land. Why is this? Cultural change is inevitably a slow process. Over 50 years we have gone from isolating the severely distressed and disabled members of our society in asylums to a policy of community integration, but the myths and stereotypes that surround 'madness' take longer to change. We as mental health workers must continue actively to support that change by challenging discrimination wherever we find it. The most important help we can give is to stand alongside people in their efforts to retain or rebuild a meaningful and valued life. We also need to take a hard look at our own attitudes – how many of us would engage with clients socially if that went beyond professional contact time? How many of us would invite them to share our interests and sources of enjoyment? I believe we have become rather fixated by the 'imperative' of maintaining boundaries. Of course there are ethical limits, but boundaries can be flexible: I have gone with clients to football matches, to the cinema, to my squash club, to my singing group, to my pub – sometimes outside designated working hours – without the professional relationship being compromised.

I find it hard to understand how psychiatry can remain so apolitical. How can we continue to treat the casualties of a society that is damaging to mental health without challenging social policy and working for social change? Could it be that somewhere in that dark paranoid vision of psychiatry as an agency of the state lies a kernel of truth that the unspoken role of psychiatry is to patholo- gise and pacify the distressed so as to mollify social malcontent!

Out of the labyrinth – a personal reflection on recovery

Anna Last

It was the year 2000 when I was first diagnosed with anorexia and clinical depression, although both had been active for a long time before. Not long after this my whole life became engulfed in mental illness and I became entirely overwhelmed and profoundly at a loss as to how best to help myself get well again. At the very depths of these illnesses I found it increasingly difficult to communicate, socialise or to leave my home which resulted in me having to give up a successful career in librarianship.

My background is rather ordinary, if somewhat privileged. I grew up in an affluent community on the Suffolk coast, a coastline that I have grown to love. I was the eldest child in our family, received a good education, enjoyed music and had many friends. At school I did well, liked studying and I subsequently went away to university to study for a geography degree. Following graduation I continued my studies in London and successfully completed my masters degree in Library and Information Studies. Then, drawn back like a marine creature by the pull of the sea, I took a librarian's post a few miles inland from my home town.

Before I became unwell I was a young enthusiastic professional commencing a career in librarianship working at a local college. I was enjoying an independent life with my own flat, returning home at weekends to visit my family. In my free time I met old friends from university, travelled and enjoyed the arts and the cinema. My future stretched out positively ahead of me and perhaps naively I expected none of this to change. Then I became unwell.

Malady

The malady creeps through my body,
Crawling through every bone.
Swimming through my veins,
Heavy in my stomach like a stone.
The parasite lives inside me,
Controlling my brain and my mind.
Dominating – at other times lying low.
Is it my friend or foe?
Without my malady I could be alive,
With my malady I hardly survive.
Go away, leave me be,
The malady and me.

The next few years were a time of trying conventional treatments available, in the hope that my symptoms would be alleviated and my recovery would commence. I tried many different antidepressants and antipsychotic drugs, yet none of these appeared to do anything, even at high doses, other than to take the edge off my anxiety and despair. There was not one drug that I could pick out and say, 'Yes that really made a difference to my life'. Treatments included electroconvulsive therapy (ECT), cognitive behavioural therapy (CBT) and other forms of psychotherapy, all of which had a limited effect on my illness. I have had 20 admissions, both voluntary and compulsory, to my local psychiatric hospital, a private hospital and a specialist eating disorders unit. All these admissions undoubtedly saved my life, yet had little influence on my illness.

Feeling increasingly frustrated that life was moving on yet I appeared to be stuck in the depths of despair, I began to experiment with strategies outside those conventional psychiatry had to offer. It was at that time that I discovered creative writing and began to use it as a self-help therapy.

Back then my understanding was that I had an illness and the illness could be treated. I did not understand that in order to recover I needed to go down into the labyrinth of my distress and would return to the light only when I had overcome what I found there. One problem had always been that in my depressed state of mind I had great difficulty communicating my distress experience to anyone, except of course through my symptoms. But once I realised that there are many other ways of communicating – art, drama, creative writing – my recovery journey could begin.

I would not describe myself as a writer. I had never before sat down purposefully to write. In a way I think writing found me, at a time when I needed to expose and release my innermost thoughts and emotions. Creative writing emerged as my own personal therapy and was so unlike the conventional therapies I had tried which had often left me feeling unheard and misunderstood.

Writing was different. I was able to explore the depths of my mind with some clarity. The page was my mentor, always there for me, available and accessible in times of distress and despair. The page can seem kinder than humans: it waits, it listens, it accepts and does not bite back and confuse me. Through writing I have begun to explore a labyrinth of secrets and fears. Everything I had suppressed and kept hidden for so long I am beginning to face, understand and accept. My battle with mental illness has become easier and instead of retreating from the world I have begun to engage with the realities of life.

My experiment with writing led to the publication of a collection of my poems called *Analgesia*. These poems were an exploration of my journey through mental illness and the act of writing them was part of my recovery process. Although very personal I wanted to share that experience with others, explaining why I am as I am today – a way of saying, this is where I got lost; this is where I found myself again.

I no longer feel as I felt when I wrote the poems and in that sense they are markers of my recovery. For me recovery is not time-specific. It had an identified beginning – momentary beginnings in my distress-filled life that seemed gradually to gather strength and momentum - and one day will have an end. Though I am not sure whether the end will mean I'm cured! My illness and recovery have felt like a painful transition during which time I have been an outcast from normal life. Now I am discovering life again, taking back control and responsibility for my life.

Reflecting on my experience of mental illness has taught me things about my life and life in general. Before I became unwell I seemed to race through life, not analysing or reflecting on the purpose and meaning of being me and being alive. Being unwell has made me stop and evaluate my life, allowing me to feel more fulfilled and satisfied. After years of daily thoughts obsessing about my death, feeling I no longer wanted to be alive, after scores of attempts to end my life, the lure of death became the lure of life. My life began to change for the better; I genuinely felt I wanted to be alive.

The place I'm in now is not the place I was in prior to my mental illness. It's different – better!

Almost

A gentle breeze blows through my hair,
Alive again I feel
My delicate lips taste the salty sea air
Alive again I feel
Soft spring sunshine warms my cheek
Alive again I feel
The grey North Sea laps at my feet
Alive again I feel
Perfect white clouds dominate blue sky
Alive again I feel.
Overhead gulls drift skilfully by
Alive again I feel
Pure white swans in salt marsh,
Alive again I feel.
Powerful light dazzles marram grass
Alive again I feel.
I know I'm leaving my cave behind
As I recognise the beauty of the coast.
The erosion of loneliness –

   I need to find

   Acceptance,

   Love and care,

   For that

   I search

   The most

(Poems from *Analgesia* published with the kind permission of the publisher and author.)

The spiritual dimension of recovery

6

*All shall be well and all
shall be well. All manner
of things shall be well.*

Julian of Norwich

Introduction

It may seem divergent to start this chapter with a quote from a 14th century mystic and anchorite; however, Julian of Norwich is well known in our time both through her own writing, 'The Revelations of Divine Love', and through the story of Margery Kempe. Kempe was a wealthy woman from Kings Lynn who began to experience visions and revelations of a religious nature which precipitated a state of emotionality, excitement and religious fervour. Her behaviour caused much censure in her local parish where her emotionally charged religious declamations were seen by some as blasphemy and by others as madness. In her confusion and alienation she consulted Julian, a woman known for her wisdom and compassion. Julian listened without judgement, validating Margery's experience and affirming her as someone blessed with Divine visitation and God's love. She did not underestimate the difficulties of the spiritual path, reportedly saying to Margery:

> *Set all your trust in God. Do not fear the language of the world, for the more the despising, shame and reprove, the more is your merit in the sight of God. Patience is necessary for you, for in that you shall keep your soul. (Cited in Thorne 1998, p. 110)*

Margery returned to her parish both calmer and strengthened by her conversation with Julian.

It does not require a great leap of imagination to see Margery as someone in the midst of an overwhelming personal and spiritual crisis. Excluded by her community, despairing and in distress, she sought comfort and guidance from a spiritual counsellor and because she was heard in a compassionate, affirming way was able to see her experience as the beginning of a spiritual odyssey and not as a sign of insanity.

For many people recovering from a troubled state of mind is synonymous with a spiritual journey, a journey that gives a greater sense of meaning and whole-ness to their lives. The spiritual quest is seldom a blissful search for a more spirit-ually conscious way of being and often comes out of an experience of confusion and despair, a state of mind which prompts us to engage in a serious reflection on our lives. To Inglesby (2004) this journey within can be seen as a pilgrim-age that begins with leaving the known and familiar world of experience and journeying into the unknown realms of the psyche to find salvation in our true selves and to reconnect with the joy of being. This is not an easy road. It is an arduous journey, but once started:

> All sorts of things occur to help one that would not otherwise have occurred. A whole stream of events issues from the decision, raising in one's favour all manner of unseen incidents and meetings and material assistance which no man could have dreamed would have come his way. Whatever you can do or dream you can do, begin it. Boldness has genius, power and magic in it. Begin it now. (Goethe cited in Inglesby 2004, p. 120)

This chapter concerns that pilgrimage.

· · · · · · · · · · ·

The soul is a metaphysical concept that does not fit easily into our rationalist culture. Yet there has never been a time in the history of humankind when the soul has not found expression in a reverence, wonderment and celebration at this paradise of which we are part. Even in today's predominantly secular soci-ety, the soul restlessly stirs within us, perhaps more urgently, for we have largely forgotten what it means to live soulfully. This discomfort expresses itself in a profound sense of meaninglessness, emptiness and disillusionment – a dispirit-ed state of mind that is endemic in our time (Moore 1994). We may seek to ease this discomfort through our materialism and hedonism, but that offers us no more than transient distraction and there is now an addictive quality to our consumerism and pleasure seeking as we desperately search for something to fill the aching void within.

In the contemporary Western lifestyle there is seldom the quietness and solitude necessary to reflect on life, to commune with the deepest parts of our humanity and to reconnect with our spiritual core. Our lives are lived in a frenetic rela-tional way, with our most intimate relationships giving meaning to our lives. We experience a strong need to exorcise the anxiety associated with the *separ-ateness of being* by merging our life with that of others. So important are rela-tionships in our lives that it is regarded as somewhat eccentric to also desire and require solitude. Storr (1988), in discussing the value and significance of soli-tude, argues that the capacity to be alone is linked with a sense of a personal life, with self-realisation, and with becoming aware of one's deepest needs, feelings and impulses. He goes further in likening the experience of solitude to the privacy of prayer – encapsulated moments of communion with God. Whether we actually pray or not, into that empty moment of inviolate peace may come a sense of oneness with divinity, sometimes only briefly but nonetheless profoundly. Such moments of meaningful solitude are captured powerfully in the biblical invocation to all seekers of the spiritual way to, 'Be still and know that I am God' (Psalm 46).

Most of our therapeutic endeavour in the face of others' distress is interpersonal and we place less value on the role of solitude in the healing process (Storr 1988). Even in psychotherapeutic sessions, ever keen to make a helpful intervention, we fail to recognise the true value to the client of being alone with himself/herself in the presence of the therapist. The therapeutic arena is first and foremost a safe, quiet space where someone can begin to process their troubled thoughts and feelings, find meaning and regain a sense of harmony. Mental hospitals, despite their dehumanising regimes, once provided a place of refuge, a retreat from the harsh realities of life and the vagaries of the mind, a place where people could find the tranquillity to reflect on their lives and regain their equilibrium. This hardly seems possible today in the 'mind factories' that many acute admission units have become. There is surely a case for every mental health facility to have a dedicated quiet space, a sanctuary, where people can spend time in unmolested solitude, enveloped in quietude.

Soul and spirit are hard to define. There is an ineffable quality about what they represent. Yet most people experience an intuitive knowing that goes beyond language when they use the terms. In a study of the nature of spiritual care in the context of mental health services conducted through a series of focus groups, Greasley et al (2001) tease out words and phrases people most often use in association with spiritual care. These are included in an overview of the language of spiritual life below (Box 6.1). They seem to me to be words that take us deeply

115

Box 6.1

The language of spiritual life

Spiritual care/interpersonal
Love; Caring; Kindness; Compassion; Grace; Companionship; Counsel; Presence

Spiritual care/practice
Prayer; Worship; Observance; Reading Religious/ Spiritual/ Inspirational Texts; Meditation; Yoga; Solitude; Quietude; Communion with Nature; Access Sacred Icons; Access Sacred Spaces; Ethical Living/Being; Retreats; Rituals; Pilgrimages

Spiritual wellbeing
Serenity; Calm; Peace; Solace; Hope; Comfort; Acceptance; Balance; Harmony; Joy; Sorrow; Fortitude; Grace

into the essence of what it means to be human, going beyond the usual scientific schemas by which we seek to define our natures. To live a more soulful or spiritual life is to be in touch with a source of benign power within all of us; a power which allows us to see more clearly, feel more deeply and know more surely.

Speaking personally, my Anglican upbringing had a profound effect on me as a young man and my thinking still continues to be filtered through layers of Christian teaching. I therefore think of being in touch with this benign power as coming closer to God or, to put it another way, of realising the divinity within us. But there are many other ways of conceptualising this, metaphysical and psycho-spiritual, unrelated to any organised religion. My own journey inward has not primarily been through a contemplative, prayerful life in any formal religious sense, but mainly through psychotherapeutic exploration. In the end it seems to me to lead to the same 'sacred place' where we come to experience the truth of our essential goodness or Godliness; a truth that extends to the whole of humanity, indeed the whole of creation. It is at the spiritual core of our being that we encounter loving kindness, compassion and peace. During those times in my life when I have been in despair, in peril of being overwhelmed by the painful vicissitudes of life, it has been returning to that place that has given me the strength to continue.

Living a more soulful life does not of course imply a life of serene joy – life brings suffering even to the most devout spiritual traveller – but it does teach forbearance in the knowledge that, even though our spirit might be overlaid by the trials of life, it is never extinguished. I am reminded of that wonderful medieval prayer that seeks to reconnect us with the Source:

> God be in my head and in my understanding
> God be in my eyes and in my looking
> God be in my mouth and in my speaking
> God be in my heart and in my thinking
> God be at my end and in my departing.

There is a recognition that psychiatry and psychology, the sciences of the mind, do not have all the answers to the disturbance and distress that assail our psyches. There is a sense that something is missing, that although our unquiet minds can be pacified and our equilibrium restored, those sciences have little to offer that will enable us to transmute or transcend suffering. It could be argued that they work against the spiritual quest for meaning and wholeness by offering the promise of answers to the problems of living in the form of neuroleptic medication and quick-fix psychotherapies. As mental health professionals we need a measure of humility – we simply do not know what is best for individuals in their anguish. We can help and people can help themselves, but what is clear is that for many people such help must have a spiritual dimension (Mental Health Foundation 2000, 2002).

Traditionally institutional religion and faith communities have been the rock that people have leaned on in adversity, distress and confusion. The comfort and help that can be accessed through places of worship, sacred texts, prayer and religious observance, clergy and the support of a faith community can be considerable. Given that compassionate care, enshrined in the story of the Good Samaritan, is surely central to the ethos of all world religions, it is always surprising when that help is not forthcoming. Sometimes, it seems as if faith communities abdicate their responsibilities for the wellbeing of a fellow member when the problem is seen as psychiatric. It is symbolic of the split that still exists in the care of mind, body, spirit, despite holism becoming a watchword of good practice in religious and secular care. Many people in confused and troubled states of mind experience a need for spiritual support but find institutional religion either unaccepting or too rigid and dogmatic in its views.

I have worked with two Christian clients over the past few years who have had very different experiences of spiritual support through the Church. One is a man with a twelve year history of episodes of being deeply troubled by voices which provide a sometimes negative, guiding commentary on his life as well as pressure of thought and feelings of guilt. This torment has at times been so intense that he has attempted to end his life. Since being drawn to the Church and embracing a Christian way of life he has been able to live with more equanimity. He attributes this to the fact that religion has given his life meaning and purpose and he now has in his life the ultimate source of wisdom and forgiveness.

The second client is man who had a deprived, deeply damaging childhood and who now experiences wild fluctuations of mood and episodes of paranoid hostility. He is a man in touch with the earthiness of human nature and with his spiritual core who has desperately sought acceptance and love and healing through the Church only to find rejection and condemnation.

It has often seemed to me that both Christianity and psychiatry have an unhelpful bias in their dogma towards a view of humankind as essentially flawed and fallen from grace. In the case of the Church people are designated as essentially sinful; in the case of secular psychiatry they are seen as driven by the unconscious to behave, in fantasy or reality, in self-gratifying, conflict-creating ways. In both cases the basic conception of humankind is one of 'badness' that requires on the one hand absolution and on the other treatment. What is so badly missing in psychiatry and in the mainstream Christian Church is a belief in the essential goodness of humankind. In the tradition of Celtic spirituality, for example, there is a belief that what is deepest in us and in all of creation is not our sinfulness but the imprint of God and the goodness of creation. If we could see ourselves as blessed with a potential for goodness rather than cursed with original sin, our sense of wellbeing and the wellbeing of the earth would be greatly enhanced.

Over the past decade there have been a number of anthologies published in which people who have experienced serious breakdowns in their mental health have described epiphanies in the midst of turmoil and experienced their recovery as a spiritual journey (Mental Health Foundation 1999; Barker et al 1999; Barker & Buchanan-Barker 2004).

Diane Webb talks about her experience of William Blake's 'Heaven in a wild flower' and describes awakening to the divine presence within her and within all of creation which for her has led to healing. Her spiritual practice is not through formal religious observance but through writing haikus 'which in the space of a single breath share moments of connectedness with other miracles of creation and celebrate the divine creativity in which we all participate' (Mental Health Foundation 1999).

Tim Harvey gains strength and comfort from the story of the Prodigal Son, from the knowledge that a return to God is always possible and that 'no treatment can replace His loving arms' (Mental Health Foundation 1999).

John Excell finds a positive dimension to the experience of schizophrenia through Joseph Campbell's observation that 'the schizophrenic is drowning in the same water that the mystic swims in with delight' (Mental Health Foundation 1999).

Vicky Nicholls, through spiritual counselling, prayer, meditation and visualisation:

> clambered up from the bottom of the journey so I saw things in a new way. After much hard work I saw that underneath my anxieties was a great pool of love and tenderness, the liquid amber under the tangle of thorns. (Mental Health Foundation 1999)

Angela Morton describes how her recovery was sustained by the iconic imagery of Christianity surfacing in her consciousness and expressing itself in poetry:

> I found my mind working and re-working the phrase 'and only when'. I was peeling potatoes when the first line came into my head – 'and only when I'd lain in severing heat', then more sentences – 'and only when I'd lain in binding ice/and only when all life and love had lain eclipsed'. I was startled to find that I was writing as if I was Lazarus speaking. (Mental Health Foundation 1999; the full text of this poem can be read at the end of this chapter)

We can see from these testimonies how the spiritual quest can take many forms and contribute significantly to the recovery process. For many people it can happen through the teachings and spiritual practice of one of the world religions, for others through the practice of yoga, meditation, contemplation and prayer, not allied to any particular faith but interfaith in nature. Sometimes spiritual consciousness develops through a growing communion and connection with the natural world. The poet E.E. Cummings expresses this evocatively and joyfully in a poem which begins 'i thank You God most for this amazing day: for the leaping greenly spirit of trees' and ends 'now the ears of my ears awake and the eyes of my eyes are opened'.

Others tap into their spiritual core through sacred dance, sacred song or chants. Often it will be found in poetry, music and art, which can act like a portal to another dimension of experience; as artist Ben Nicholson wrote, 'As I see it, art and religion are the same thing' (cited in Hardy 1979). Housden (2003), in an inspiring anthology, talks about poetry which can:

> give voice to a spiritual reality that is beyond the copyright of any religion. It voices longings of the spirit and our deep desires – the desire for meaning, for a life of passion and creativity, for a sense of belonging, for wisdom and as always for love.

There has been a growing interest in the connection between mystical experiences and other extraordinary states of consciousness sometimes diagnosed as psychotic. Many people have experiences of altered states of reality which they interpret in a religious/spiritual way. Thirty years ago Professor Alister Hardy and colleagues at the Religious Experience Research Unit in Oxford collected over 4000 testimonies of deeply felt transcendental experiences (Hardy 1979). The research indicated the ubiquitous nature of such experiences which can take many forms, have many triggers and raise awareness of a 'benevolent non-physical power'.

Common among these accounts are extraordinary sensory experiences that are perceived as spiritual in nature: voices guiding or calming; the experience of being spoken through; a revelatory or transformative experience of light; a sense of being physically touched in some unaccountable way that is felt to be healing or comforting. Other frequently reported experiences are more affective in nature. These include enveloping moments of security and peace; of joy; of new strength; of inspiration or guidance; of hope and optimism; a feeling of love; of unity with one's surroundings; a sense of forgiveness, restoration and renewal; a sense of presence. These experiences were often fleeting in nature but remained vividly in the memory and in many cases had a transformative effect on the individual's life. Sometimes, but by no means always, they occurred in the context of some kind of personal/emotional crisis but, as Hardy points out, this does not necessarily invalidate them as spiritual experiences. He concluded from his research that there was good evidence for a transcendental/spiritual reality; a feeling that 'something other' can be sensed 'beyond the conscious self, with which the individual can have communion in one way or another – whether spoken of as God or not'.

The following testimony illustrates the powerful healing nature of some religious experience:

> Gradually I became more psychotic and attempted suicide. I had done something which I considered utterly dreadful and I was being driven to self-destruction by an intense feeling of guilt. I had only one desire – to be forgiven. In hospital I was seen by psychiatrists and the chaplain and my family but I was unable to communicate sensibly with any of them. Then quite dramatically the whole picture changed overnight. The weight of guilt had been lifted and I was myself again, quite rational and ready to go home. This recovery was not due to any medical intervention and the psychiatrist and the priest were at a loss to understand this transformation. But it was to me quite simple – God had forgiven me. It was not a temporary healing; I have never needed treatment since that time. (Cited in Hardy 1979, p. 60)

Is it possible to differentiate between manifestations of the ego as pseudo mystical states and authentic revelatory experience? Miranda Holden, director of the Interfaith Seminary in London, argues that truth as opposed to illusion is revealed in the fact that a transpersonal experience always brings a person closer to the heart of God (Holden 2005). It is felt as deeply loving and peaceful and is a source of loving kindness towards others. It is always orientated towards unity, guiding the individual in the direction of forgiveness, healing and integration. Out of authentic spiritual experiences 'right speech' and 'right action' spring. People are often fired with intentionality following such experiences and are moved to act in transformative ways. Holden suggests that it is possible to check the truth and meaning of any revelatory experience by simply asking. Guidance and confirmation will always be given in some form if we remain open to it.

Romme & Escher (1993, 2000), in their groundbreaking work on voice hearing, point to many examples of individuals, both with and without a psychiatric history, who experience their voices in a spiritual/mystical way or as some form of extrasensory perception, and for whom orthodox psychiatric interpretations just do not ring true. Many people have what they describe as 'inner voice experiences' which they see as a guiding mentor that shapes their life and spiritual development; others, who have a clearer sense of voices as being external and not of themselves, regard them as more mystical–divine 'showings'. In other cases voices are experienced as a psychic phenomenon. As with all voices, whether of psychiatric significance or not, what is important is how they are understood, coped with and integrated into the individual's life, which is a process aided by being able to confide openly with others who are accepting and appropriately responsive.

A remarkable client I have had some contact with in the last few years is a young woman who lives much of her life among a 'community of voices'. Many of these voices are derogatory but others have more of a psychic feel to them in that they are the voice of her dead mother and sometimes the voices of dead babies. The approach to working with her voices has been a fairly orthodox one – partly symptomatic, treating her with neuroleptic medication which she takes intermittently, and partly by helping her find strategies for coping with her voices. Neither has provided much relief. She can sometimes ignore the voices enough to engage with others on a rational plane but occasionally they are so persistent and intrusive that she is totally distracted.

Recently, however, there has been an effort to look at the spiritual side of her voice hearing experience and their meaning for her. Although not currently a practising member her spiritual upbringing is rooted in the Pentecostal Church where a belief in the intrusion of spirit entities, both good and evil, into our earthly lives is accepted. At times it seems as if these good and bad entities manifest themselves as voices and have vociferous debates about her virtue or lack of it. It is a debate in which she often interjects angrily but which she feels powerless to stop. She is desperate for a child and believes that the voices of the babies she hears are her own children who have been stolen from her because they were not conceived in love but in lust. Her mother's voice admonishes her for her 'wayward', 'unpenitent' life just as she did when she was alive. To discuss her voice hearing experiences in these terms gives them meaning and allows a more empowered attitude towards them to grow.

What is crucial is for mental health professionals to be receptive, accepting and responsive to the spiritual needs of clients. The spiritual and religious realm of experience may be difficult for clients to talk about precisely because they are unsure of how it will be received. The fear is that it will be disregarded or worse pathologised; as one survey respondent put it: 'To invalidate a person's spirituality no matter how distorted it is, is to invalidate the real core sense of self and I think once you do that you risk doing untold damage to somebody' (Mental Health Foundation 2002).

Research by Macmin & Foskett (2004) suggests that beyond the comfort of an empathic interaction the main reason for talking about spiritual and religious experience is a search for meaning. Although a small scale project, it helpfully illuminates the interface between spirituality and mental health problems. The researchers conclude that when people are heard and their spiritual life acknowledged:

> their own religious resources began to emerge and their breakdowns became breakthroughs. They encountered parts of themselves which they did not know existed and which helped them make sense of their crises. They spoke of the power of humour, healing, blessing, inspiration, prayer, compassion, salvation, faith, inner change and the value of sacred places and spaces both within mental health services and in the community. (p. 35)

The search for meaning and purpose is an important motivating force in all our lives. In the secular world it is found, if it is found at all, in a cherished family life, in the worthwhileness of our work, in a creative life, or in selfless activity for the greater good. It often seems to me that something or someone to recover for, beyond oneself, is a missing stimulus for many people who seem stuck in their recovery journey. It may well be that people need to be their own 'worthwhile project'. Recognising their own virtue and value may be a starting point, but when they feel connected to 'something greater than themselves, some ideal that will lift them beyond everyday struggles, a new motivation flows inside them which can carry them through difficulties with unerring purposefulness' (Van Deurzen-Smith 1988).

Existential philosophy is centrally concerned with the issue of meaninglessness, which is seen by Victor Frankl (2004) as the paramount cause of life crises. Beyond the concerns of everyday reality are the beliefs, aspirations, values, and ideals that give meaning to our life. Many people find *cosmic meaning* in a belief in God and see life's purpose as fulfilling the Divine Will by living according to scriptural teachings. Of course, not everyone of faith has such a fundamentalist view and there are many versions of what a divinely inspired life means.

Existentialism rejects the belief in a divinely inspired life and proposes the secular view that we alone have the responsibility for searching out and giving our lives meaning. For some people this search for meaning leads to altruistic action, to work that is of service to others, makes the world a better place to live or contributes to a cause for the greater good. This gives life its sense of worthwhileness. For some, creativity – not just in the arts but in diverse human activity such as science, teaching, homemaking – gives life meaning. It has been suggested that many artistically inclined people are keenly sensitive to 'cosmic indifference' – the essential meaninglessness of life – and find creative endeavour a powerful antidote. A more nihilistic position resonates for a great many people who see no meaning in life other than to live it and live it fully. Yalom (1980) puts it this way:

> The purpose of life from this view, is simply to live fully, to retain one's sense of astonishment at the miracle of life, to plunge oneself into the natural rhythm of life, and to search for pleasure in the deepest possible sense.

Humanistic psychology has added to the debate about the meaning of human existence, by stressing the imperative for personal wellbeing and social accord, of actualising our potential as human beings. This quest has provided a purpose and meaning for existence to many people in Western society over the past 50 years. Although it has been widely criticised as a manifesto for the self-obsessed, to see it in such a way is a distortion. Abraham Maslow, one of the founding fathers of the human potential movement, argued powerfully that the opposite is true: that self-actualisation leads inevitably to a more transcendent way of being. The more we move towards self-realisation, the more positive values such as 'kindness, honesty, love, courage, goodness, selflessness and serenity' express themselves in an orientation towards the wellbeing of others and our world (cited in Yalom 1980).

Questions of spirituality and meaning may be difficult issues to grapple with but they are ones we need to engage with if we are to create a service that is truly in the business of recovering mental health. If we aspire to become holistic practitioners we must first of all be prepared to ask ourselves searching questions about our own beliefs, about what gives our own lives meaning. This could and should be facilitated in the context of multidisciplinary educational programmes on the spiritual dimension of care and recovery.

Sadly, much of what is currently held up as gold standard practice in evidence-based psychiatry is reductive, offering only the crudest understanding of what it means to be human. As Barker & Buchanan-Barker (2004) eloquently put it:

> The richness of our imagination and the sheer breadth of our emotions – stretching from tragic farce to heavenly bliss – are largely ignored. Certainly our instinct to fulfil ourselves in a wide variety of ways and achieve a sense of connection with the wider universe of consciousness is missed in its entirety. We might well argue that, viewed from a holistic perspective, the old psychology that underpins

psychiatry and much mental health work is less than human ignoring our cap-
acity for everyday genius, our inherent complexity and eccentricity, and our sense
of soulfulness. (p. 223)

Spikenard and jasmine
and only when I'd lain in severing heat:
and only when I'd lain in binding ice:
and only when all life and love had lain eclipsed:
and only when my sister's tears had lain,
    dissolving in my hair:
and only when their linen had been bound about my bones:
and only when I had been borne along the lonely path:
and only when the stone had sealed the tomb:

and only when the binding cloth unwound:

and only when I was made whole again:
    and by the river, unremembering,
I'd walked again, had walked among birdsong
    and perfumed flowers,
had walked in the valley among the spikenard and jasmine:
only then Lord, did I hear you call my name.

Angela Morton

(Reproduced with the kind permission of the Mental Health Foundation)

The creative dimension of recovery

7

*Every artist might not be a
special kind of person,
but every person is a special
kind of artist.*

Eric Gill

Introduction

Creativity is a defining characteristic of what it means to be human. Through-out history human beings have sought to express themselves in aesthetic ways, ways that express the wonder and reverence for the world in which we live, the complexity of what it is to be human. The urge to create is a primal urge that struggles to find expression in today's pre-packaged Western consumer culture. So much of the art that is valued today is 'gallery art', a product rather than a deeply personal statement. There seems little room for 'raw art' – art that is not bound by convention or reason but is a spontaneous expression of an inner vision. Outsider art and writing that is created by untutored yet gifted artists in the process of their recovery is of this nature: a raw authentic self-expression that powerfully documents their journey. It is no coincidence that we feel ener-gised and alive when we are deeply involved in some creative project. Creativity is linked with spontaneity, innovation, imagination, intuition, emotion, playful-ness, meaning and soulfulness and as such is central to our wellbeing.

Creativity is of course not simply expressed through the arts but in many facets of our working and personal lives. Fundamentally it is seen in the creation of ourselves. As Carl Rogers has shown in his lifelong study of the 'emergent self', given *the core conditions* for growth, we are in a continuing state of *becoming a person*; recreating ourselves in ways that reveal more of our authentic self, less bound by the conditions of selfhood imposed by others (Rogers 1961). Much suffering and distress results from repressing our creative urge to grow as individuals and under the pressures of social expectation and conformity the growing edge of our personalities fails to flourish. Abraham Maslow claimed that what we regard as psychologically normal is really the 'psychopathology of the average', so underdeveloped is our human potential (cited in Egan 2002).

Theologian Mathew Fox argues that we each of us have a spark of divinity within, which gifts us the power of creation, the power to recreate ourselves and our world, to fuse the chaotic, disparate, jarring parts of our personalities into a more harmonious whole (Fox 2002). As we shall see in this chapter, art and the creative life are, for many people, integral to healing and wellbeing.

• • • • • • • • • • •

The mental suffering of many of our great poets, writers, composers and artists, documented in numerous biographies, gives some substance to the commonly held belief that creativity and 'madness' are often intertwined. Simply casting a net among the writers and poets of the last century whose state of mind was sufficiently troubled to require an admission to a psychiatric hospital reveals how many suffered for their art. Among this group are Robert Lowell, Anne Sexton, Sylvia Plath, Eugene O'Neill, Virginia Woolf, Tennessee Williams, Ernest Hemingway, F. Scott Fitzgerald, T.S. Eliot. For many artists the travails of human life resonate deeply within them and they live their lives exposed more than most to the tidal flow of joys and sorrows. This of course provides inspiration for so much of the music, art and writing that we value, but it comes at some cost. Studies show that suicide rates among writers and artists are 16 times higher than the expected rate in the general population and for severe mood disorders they are eight to ten times higher (Jamison 1993). Art that has the power to transfix us with its beauty and meaning is created along the tide line between reason and unreason, a place where passions flow freely, where reality and convention shift and great dreams are thrown up. But artists who do not have a secure foothold on the shores of reason can be swept away by the inrushing and outflowing tides.

Not only does art 'etched from pain' give creative work its power but it also offers an escape from anguish. Graham Greene observed that 'writing is a form of therapy; sometimes I wonder how all those who do not write, compose or paint can mange to escape the madness, the melancholia, the panic and fear which is inherent in the human condition'. Kay Redfield Jamison (1993), in her extraordinary analysis of creativity and manic depressive illness, captures the notion of art as therapy, observing that:

> creative work can act not only as a means of escape from pain but also as a way of structuring chaotic feelings and thoughts, numbing pain through abstraction and the rigours of disciplined thought and creating a distance from the source of despair. (p. 123)

Psychiatrist and analyst Anthony Storr, in an exploration of the dynamics of creative acts, talks about the healing function of art in states of deep sadness

126

and melancholia. 'Writing and other creative activities can be a way of coping with loss, whether that be some current bereavement or the feelings of emptiness and loss that accompany severe depression' (Storr 1988, p. 128).

Storr suggests that because creative skill is an attribute highly valued by society, many creative people seek to replenish their self-esteem through the appreciation of their work received from others. But for many, any such acclaim soon evaporates and only a faint emotional trace may linger in the psyche. This may explain, in part, why many artists are driven in pursuit of their vocation and prone to recurrent crises of confidence and self-worth. Many artists, vulnerable to depression, are people who have abandoned hope of ever being loved and prized for themselves and instead channel their real self, along with their unmet need for approbation, into their work. To then have that work criticised as having little worth can therefore be experienced as an enormous psychological blow. It is this dynamic that can sometimes lead to a creative block. If people feel that their creative work, invested with so much of themselves, will never be good enough and will be rejected, then it is small wonder that some creative work is never completed.

Creative expression allows people to communicate, often in symbolic or metaphorical form, feelings, thoughts and perceptions that cannot be expressed verbally. The artist is able to use his or her talent to capture and express, in a controlled way, feelings that disturb and threaten to overwhelm the psyche and beyond that find meaning in them. Cathy Conroy, a powerful and creative voice in the advocacy movement in Australia, is someone who has written evocatively about her journey through, but not beyond, her experience of psychosis (Conroy 1999). She recognises creative potential in her breakdown and is in no doubt that her life would be diminished without 'its current depth and intensity, having to forever tame my feelings and smooth the rush and ache of my heart'. She describes the importance of creative expression in discovering meaning and value in distressed disturbed states of mind, recalling that in her early hospitalisation:

> collage was important to my recovery. It seemed to offer me clarity as I ripped pictures from magazines assembling the fragments of photos and illustrations in a way that encapsulated my inner experience. The fragments formed symbols of my psychic world, emerging from the depths of inner caverns. The meanings I attributed have remained very important to me in understanding the patterns of my life contributing to my health and my illness. (p. 65)

We are familiar with the cliché of the rebellious artist and, although a clichéd image, it contains some psychological truth. In order to find themselves, many people have to rebel against their past, their parents and all they have stood for. If an individual's emergent self has not been lovingly nurtured and prized and their predominant experience was of coldness or rejection, then it is likely that a legacy of anger and hostility will remain in their psyche to fuel their acts of rebellion. It is unsurprising therefore that this emotionally charged rebelliousness should find its way into a person's art or writing which may be highly original and defy convention. For that work to be lauded mitigates some of the guilt or anxiety the artist feels about the potential destructiveness of their feelings.

There is also something important about the harmony of a painting, a poem or music which has the power to quieten and order the troubled mind, allowing the individual to encounter a unity and wholeness that has been lost or eluded them in their lives. Storr (1972), in reflecting on this psychological function of art, argues 'that the greater the disharmony within, the greater the spur to seek harmony, or if one has the gifts, to create harmony'. As Tennyson, who suffered bouts of severe depression throughout his life, wrote: 'But for the unquiet heart and brain/A use in measured language lies'.

After my son's suicide his portfolio was found to contain an extensive series of untitled abstract paintings which have since been exhibited to much acclaim. Some of these are shown on the back cover of this book. The persistence with which he returned to the creative task of juxtaposing these irregular forms and variant colours suggests now an urgent need to solve a problem. In a review of his exhibition, the reviewer comments that

> in every painting there is an attempt to create a sense of harmony and balance from what is potentially disharmonious, and in most cases he succeeds, but there are some paintings where tension and incipient confusion bear the marks of the struggle involved. As his depression tightened its grip and his view on the world took on a more ominous perspective, he found it increasingly difficult to paint and was thus deprived of a source of relief and resolution.

I live with many of his paintings now and I find in them the struggles we all face to keep our inner and outer worlds in some kind of balance, confronted as we are so often by potentially destabilising pressures. In much of his work there is a vibrant unity and the suggestion of something beyond, as the eye is taken to a 'window' that appears in many of the paintings. Despite the tragic culmination of his life he has left us with paintings that are full of hope.

There can be little doubt that creativity in its various forms has a role to play in recovery. A survey of 400 people using mental health services found that 45% had some experience of creative therapies/activities in the context of their care and recovery and found them *helpful or helpful at times* (Mental Health Foundation 2000). In reflecting on the beneficial elements of their creative experience respondents mentioned several factors:

- The act of creating is meaningful and satisfying in itself and can engender self-worth and a sense of achievement – as one respondent said tellingly about the value of creative expression, 'It's being able to leave your mark'.
- Creative activity is often experienced as absorbing and distracting. It necessitates an emotional and mental disengagement from a troubled and distressing internal world and thereby provides, if only temporarily, some relief.

'Focusing all my tension on a painting cleared all this crap from my head. Nothing else does it for me. I need something totally absorbing ... It blocks out the 'what ifs', the anxiety, that perpetual conversation... it blocks it out. It disappears into the mist'.

- In contrast to the above, for some people creative expression was a way of communicating disturbing and overwhelming feelings and thoughts. A chaotic troubled inner world externalised and contained in painting or writing can provide a sense of release and calm. As a contributor to this book has written: 'The listening page can seem kinder than another person. It doesn't bite back or confuse me. Through writing I'm able to uncover and explore a maze of hidden secrets, a labyrinth of uncomfortable emotions.'

- The sense of community found in a creative group can be an important healing factor. Belonging, being accepted, and as one person described to me a 'feeling of being borne back into life by the creative flow of the group', are all important recovery experiences for people who feel alienated.

- For some people art in its myriad forms can be the most therapeutic factor in their recovery, as one respondent to the Mental Health Foundation survey starkly put it, 'Art, in a nutshell, has kept me alive!'

A number of innovative arts projects have developed in Britain which enable people to be 'borne back into life by the creative flow'. Survivors' Poetry is one such example of a creative forum in which people can articulate in a poetic form their personal experiences of distress; of surviving the psychiatric system – and of coming through. Survivors' Poetry now has over 2000 members and 28 groups nationwide which hold regular workshops and perform and publish members' poetry. One member describes how at a time when he was feeling 'lost and bewildered' in an 'isolated, pointless life' he found salvation in Survivors' Poetry:

> *My* raison d'être *became very much centred on the hopes and aspirations afforded me by Survivors' Poetry. It was a vital experience to be able to share with others who were also struggling to find some meaning in their lives, which the world looks on at best as failed and at worst a burden on society. To find your words are not greeted with dismissive silence or patronising advice. To find instead that people recognise and appreciate the pain behind your experience; who value your expression as poetry and are prepared to encourage you to refine it.*

He talks about the major task of overcoming a fear of schizophrenia and how voices have been not merely the result of a biochemical imbalance but have reflected a 'deep need to find myself', a process in which Survivors' Poetry (www.survivorspoetry.com) has had a significant role (Hambrook 2000).

Another innovative example of the arts in mental health is the Mental Fight Club (MFC), a creative project that takes its name and inspiration from the art and poetry of William Blake. MFC organises events – 'happenings' – that seek to remove the 'mind forged manacles' and release the creative energies and talents of people, many of whom have lived tumultuous lives as outsiders amid the visions and voices of another reality, as Blake himself did. It now has over 500 members, half of whom have direct experience of severe mental illness.

MFC aims to raise awareness of mental wellbeing, mental distress and mental illness through openness about the inner and outer world of experience and the connectedness of all humanity in the flow of that experience. It seeks to assist in the recovery journey through group working and the development of each individual's potential, realised through participating in Mental Fight Club events. Two major events are staged annually which take the form of exhibitions, lectures, readings, installations or performances exploring the concept of 'mental fight' in all facets of life. St George, the patron saint of England, has provided a powerful motif for recent MFC events as a heroic slayer of 'dragons' wherever they are found. A current project is to stage performances of Ben Okri's epic poem 'Mental Fight', a poem which is an inspiring wake-up call to us as individuals and to all of humanity to seize the moment to 'Open up the magic casement/ Of the human spirit/ Onto a more shining world' (www.into.org. uk/mentalfightclub).

Start is an award winning arts in mental health project based in Manchester, using art as a tool in recovery from severe and enduring mental health problems (www.startmc.org.uk). Students access courses in ceramics, textiles, painting, drawing, photography and gardening, delivered by a team of artists in an affirming, empowering way. The needs and interests of individual students, not their skill level, are the key criteria for enrolment in the programme, which makes Start courses highly inclusive. In discussing the Start model, lead artist Mary Teall comments that many students begin with low self-expectation and confidence but as they become immersed in the excitement of the creative process and their engagement deepens, they are encouraged and challenged to set personal goals and build a wide portfolio of transferable skills, with personal and cognitive development taking place alongside the development of artistic and technical skills (Teall 2003).

Two Start students, who generously share their testimonies below, were able to rebuild their confidence and self-esteem and find themselves after experiencing severe mental health problems. Start allowed the students to actualise more of their potential and opened up opportunities so that their breakdowns led to very positive breakthroughs.

Caty's story

When I found the art room in the hospital I found a haven. It was a way of channelling the little energy and control I had into something positive. Then after a second hospital admission I was told about Start; that was about eight years ago. Start has helped me rebuild my self-confidence and self-belief after illness. My friendship with other Start students has helped me realise that my illness need not be a negative experience but one that is valuable to me personally and to others. I feel accepted for who I am and what I can share, and this extends beyond illness and into life experiences. I suppose you could say that Start helped me find a sense of myself.

(Reproduced with kind permission of Start in Manchester)

Aileen's story

Once I could hardly get out of bed in the mornings. Now I feel as if I have taken control of my life. Studying art at Start has boosted my confidence. I came to feel more positive about myself. I've got something to talk to people about now. Also I can talk more freely about my illness. There was a time when I was so ashamed about having a mental illness but I don't feel that anymore because it became an opportunity for me rather than something to hide. I never would have achieved what I have without falling ill and coming to Start. I know I have succeeded at things I never would have dreamt of, and that I will go on achieving more in the future.

(Reproduced with kind permission of Start in Manchester)

A recent exhibition, the Voyager Exhibition, emerged out of a research linked course which studied the work of the 'naïve' Cornish painter Alfred Wallis, himself an 'outsider artist' whose work achieved much acclaim. An appreciation of his life and work provided not only a stimulus for students' own art work but also promoted critical thinking, verbal and written expression and self-exploration. One student whose sense of identity was positively affected by the course said, 'The course made me realise I'm an artist too'. Another student who gained significantly in confidence said simply but tellingly, 'The course helped me come out from under'.

An evaluative study of outcomes for students engaged in the Alfred Wallis project shows that in addition to gaining new artistic skills, there were significant gains in social skills, cognitive abilities, emotional literacy and self-perception, which in turn promoted self-confidence, self-esteem and self-actualisation (Teall & Tortora 2004; Teall et al 2005). The outcomes were seen as adding to the evidence for art as a 'catalyst for personal development' with personal growth and change shown to be sustained well beyond the life of the project and resulting in a 'lasting sense of self transformation'.

Inside Out is a creative arts community in Ipswich established by Jan Addison and Peter Watkins for people who have experienced periods of disabling distress in their lives and who are at various stages in their recovery (www.inside outcommunity.com). Members meet weekly to explore their creativity in relation to various art forms. Local artists lead workshops in painting and drawing, printmaking, singing, creative writing, drama, sculpture and photography. The fusion of creative energy when the group meets flows into imaginative and inspired work, much of which is shown to the public at the community's annual exhibition.

The philosophy of Inside Out is that creative energy and ability are latent human characteristics that frequently get stifled by repeated critical judgment in our formative years. Many people have been told they cannot sing and have lost their voice; many people have had their art disregarded and are now unable to 'make their mark'. At Inside Out work is never judged; any authentic expression of artistic endeavour is prized. We align ourselves with 'roots' poetry, art and music – untutored creative acts that arise irrepressibly in traditional low technology cultures.

A strongly held belief that underpins the work of Inside Out is that the creative act strengthens the human spirit. When we are being creative we are using all our faculties and are more fully alive. The creative energy that stirs within us is then available for everyday living. To believe in yourself as a creative person is to walk more boldly through life. Just as making that first mark on a blank canvas, writing the first word on an empty page, singing the first note into the silent air, are beginnings that can lead to a stunning image, a moving poem, or a liberating song, so we can be artists in the way we create and recreate our own lives. Within the community, now in its fourth year, people discover and develop their artistic talents, grow in self-esteem and confidence, experience a sense of inclusion and belonging and begin to live with more hope and freedom.

Artists have an important role in society in shining a light into the dark byways of the human psyche where we may find ourselves lost and alone. In the words of the visionary poet Rainer Maria Rilke (cited in Astley 2002):

> *Art cannot be helpful through trying to help and specifically concerning ourselves with the distresses of others; but in so far as we bear our own distresses more passionately, we may give, now and then, a clearer meaning to endurance, and develop for ourselves a means of expressing the suffering within us and its conquest more precisely and clearly than is possible to those who have to apply their powers to something else.*

Recovery relationships

8

*People should not
consider so much
what they are to do,
as what they are to be.*

Meister Eckhart

Introduction

As we have seen, people who are in recovery often talk of significant turning points that changed the direction of their lives from breakdown and disintegration to breakthrough and reintegration. This often seems to involve another person being able to relate to them in a way that is enabling, a way of relating that nurtures hopefulness, self-determination and a sense of personal agency – as Patricia Deegan (1988) memorably puts it, 'a loving invitation to be something more'.

Psychiatry has absorbed from Western medicine the 'intervention imperative' – something must be done to fix what has gone wrong. As mental health professionals we can get so caught up in assessment, formulation and problem solving in the psychobiological or psychosocial sphere of an individual's life that we lose sight of the person and in doing so reinforce their sense of helplessness, perplexity and passivity. The person seeking help then starts to feel as if they are at the mercy of overwhelming biological or emotional forces beyond their comprehension and begins to act like a helpless victim, dependent on 'expert' help (Breggin 1996). If we can be more mindful of the person, be with them in the distress and chaos of their lives, be respectful of their resourcefulness, their strengths and dreams, then they will begin the journey towards a way of being in the world that is less problematic and distressing and more fulfilling. Healing is not a process that can be imposed from the outside – it always has to come from within. This chapter explores the nature of recovery relationships; how others can be those all important mentors and companions as people reconstruct their identity and their lives.

. . . .

A common theme in the testimonies of people who have transcended their vulnerabilities and disabilities is the central importance of a significant other in their recovery journey:

'Someone who believed in me at a time when I couldn't believe in myself.'
(Fisher & Deegan 1999)

'Someone who saw beneath my madness and into my potential.' (Coleman 1999)

'The best professionals involved in my care have walked alongside me, opening
themselves to the mystery that is schizophrenia. They have gained my trust,
sharing and supporting my inner search for meaning and understanding of self in
relation to illness.' (Champ 1999)

'I needed someone who would just be there – solid, non judging, not trying to force
me to do this or that, just being with me, helping me make sense of some very
frightening, but also some very beautiful and visionary experiences. My essential
need was to be grounded, connected to life and the world, not excluded and
punished.' (Cited in the British Psychological Society Report 2000)

What emerges from these interpersonal experiences, which seem to be widely shared, is that relationships which facilitate recovery are characterised by:

- An attitude of hopefulness when a person cannot be hopeful for themselves
- A belief in the capacity of people to actualise more of their potential
- A respect for and valuing of a person's subjective experience
- A collaborative enquiry into the meaning of a distress experience
- A respect for the personhood of the individual
- An acknowledgement of a person's strengths and qualities rather than a narrow focus on deficits and problems
- A shared search for the richer narrative of a person's life rather than a focus on the dominant problem laden narrative
- A respect for a person's right to self-determination which encourages self-empowerment and self-efficacy
- A recognition of the normalcy and humanity of experiences rather than the pathology.

What kind of helping, healing relationship is likely to value these attributes and allow them to flourish? In my view this is exemplified by the person-centred model of helping developed by Carl Rogers in his psychotherapeutic practice, writing and research over 40 years (Kirschenbaum & Henderson 1990). His is a philosophy of personal and social transformation that has been substantiated and advanced by exponents in America and Western Europe since his death in 1987 (Brazier 1993; Mearns & Thorne 2000). Rogers was not talking about a therapeutic technique but about a way of being that is compassionate, loving, empathic and accepting. A way of relating that prizes the humanity of the other, believing deeply in their potential. This is not something that can be turned on and off – that would imply a contrived, inauthentic way of relating. Rather it becomes part of who we are and manifests in all our relationships. Despite its ubiquity, the person-centred approach to helping is frequently misunderstood, being often seen as the relational background against which 'real therapy' or 'problem solving' takes place. This misses the point that the relationship is the therapy – it is the *relational depth* that provides the safety in which suffering can be faced and healing and growth can take place (Mearns & Thorne 2000).

The basic tenets of person-centred helping can be summed up as:

- People are okay though they might need some help recognising it
- People know what they need though they might need some help expressing it
- People can discover their own meanings though they might need some help doing it
- People can take responsibility for themselves, though they might need encouragement to take it. (Watkins 2001)

Rogers claimed there was a parallel between his relational approach to helping and what Martin Buber called the *I–Thou* relationship and this was debated in a fascinating meeting between the two men in 1957 (Kirschenbaum & Henderson 1990). Buber believed that most everyday human encounters were characterised by I–It attitudes, by which he meant that there is a tendency to objectify people and not to relate to them as persons. He saw humankind as essentially social beings, and life – in the sense of being fully alive – as depending on *open dialogues,* which allow us to feel a sense of mutual connectedness, rather than differentness and alienation. In *I–Thou* encounters there is an implicit recognition of a shared humanity, an equality and a joyful, respectful attitude towards the other (Kaufmann & Buber 1970). It is only from this position of equality that we can strive to bring order out of chaos, help others recover confidence in their humanness and *seek something of a resurrection* by returning people to emotional and social life from a position of deadness (Silver et al 2004).

Buber's concept of relating in a more spiritual way has informed the literature on helping and healing over many years, but is a long way from becoming a deeply held belief underpinning dialogues between mental health professionals and people seeking help. This is partly because the culture of the mental health system has institutionalised power differences and its whole *raison d'être* is based on the erroneous polarisation of the mad and the sane. It may be that the tenor of Buber's philosophy can never be lived out fully in professionalised helping relationships where equality and reciprocity cannot be fully realised and it is this experience which leads many people to seek supportive relationships with survivors and others in recovery, finding in those relationships the necessary allies for their recovery journey. As a user-led research report into strategies for living comments:

Having experiences in common means you are likely to feel more equal in those relationships, can ask for support and know that there will be opportunities to return it. As a consequence you do not feel so inadequate or needy. (Mental Health Foundation 2000)

De-professionalised care

It is clear that people who experience periods of disabling distress and disturbance in their lives do not necessarily need the assistance of mental health professionals in order to recover. Personal relationships, family relationships, friendships and a sense of community with others in recovery can be emotionally sustaining and empowering. Many people, who experience states of psychological overwhelm that may for a period of time incapacitate them and disrupt their life remain integrated and supported within their family and social group and find that restorative. For others, where family relationships have been fractured, where friendships and social connections have become tenuous, a protracted period of distress and disturbance can lead to further isolation and a desperate feeling of alienation and loneliness. This is a situation which does nothing to heal the heart and soul.

Many people in this alienated group meet their social and emotional needs and find a sense of belonging in alternative 'accepting communities' such as projects and programmes run by service users themselves. These take many forms: advocacy programmes, drop in resource centres, safe houses, support groups. The thread connecting what has become an international initiative is an adherence to certain basic principles: firstly they are run by people who have themselves received mental health services; they are based on a model of peer support rather than professional expertise; and they strive to minimise hierarchy, valuing the contribution of every participant (Chamberlin 2004). The affiliation and warm acceptance people find there contrasts starkly with stigmatisation and rejection by the wider community and provides some people with a surrogate family network. Valuable as these communities are, there is a danger of 'ghettoisation' and the possibility of people being trapped in socially marginalised lives. There needs to be sufficient cultural impetus within each alternative community to foster a sense of empowerment and confidence that would enable an individual to choose a more inclusive life in the wider community (Mental Health Foundation 2000).

In a reflection on her own recovery from psychosis and the trauma of hospitalisation, Foner (1996) describes the value of co-counselling in her healing. Similarly Parker (1999) describes how 'co-counselling kept me out of the psychiatric system and helped me be more effective in my life'. In this approach to helping and healing, trained co-counselling partners, who may both be people using mental health services, share the time equally, offering their partners free attention and ways of exploring distress laden experience which has resulted in a psychiatric crisis. Co-counselling theory holds that unhelpful patterns of behaviour, including psychotic symptoms, build up around the emotional legacy of past traumas, losses and adversity. If these feelings can be safely discharged, then the cause becomes open to re-evaluation and the wounded psyche begins to heal. While this conception of psychological healing is shared by most therapeutic models, what is different is the degree of trust in individuals to manage the healing process themselves within the egalitarian structure of a co-counselling session.

The Soteria project was a widely influential, drug free alternative to the conventional pharmacologically centred mental health system, established in the San Francisco area between 1971 and 1983 (Mosher 1999). At it its heart was a de-professionalised approach to helping and healing in which 'caregivers' were 'selected and trained to relate to and understand madness without preconceptions, labels, categories, judgements or the need to do anything to change, control, suppress or invalidate the experience of psychosis' (Mosher 2004, p. 32). The focus was on creating a respectful, hopeful, containing, empowering social milieu in which diagnostic labelling and antipsychotic medication were seen as impediments to recovery. The experience of psychosis was seen as a personal or developmental crisis that had meaning in the context of the current and historical life events of the person seeking help. The role of 'caregivers' was not to 'do therapy' but to be with people in their distress and perplexity in a non-intrusive, accepting, empathic way so that the meaningfulness of the crisis experience could emerge. Shared meaning was distilled not solely from an individual's subjective world but also from the interactive experience with caregivers. In that sense it is similar to the 'living learning experience', the key element in emotional healing in therapeutic communities.

Mosher identifies factors that are predictive of a positive outcome in recovery programmes:

- The presence of a perceived healing context, which could be a hospital unit, a sanctuary, a survivor led resource centre, or a community based recovery team
- Confiding relationships with helpers developed in a social context in which the barriers to the development of collaborative relationships are removed
- The gradual evolution of a shared, meaningful explanation of the crisis experience
- The therapeutic culture transmitting a positive expectation of recovery
- The recovery process creating opportunities for experiencing success.

Despite the substantial research evidence emerging from this and similar contemporary projects that psychosocial approaches are at least as effective as drug-based hospital treatment in promoting recovery across a range of symptomatic and social criteria, such approaches have been swept away in the continuing search for a magic bullet and have only played a peripheral role in the psychiatric treatment of severe mental health problems (Mosher 2004). In recent years, however, the concepts of care and recovery that were at the heart of Soteria have resurfaced in early intervention programmes and in the philosophy that underpins recovery-orientated services.

In spite of the difficulties inherent in professional helping relationships, my experience is that mental health workers can and do engage with people in meaningful ways that allow the expression of the values that both Rogers and Buber regarded as essential for the reduction of human suffering and the facilitation of growth and change. There is awareness of the need to remove a prevailing sense of hierarchy from the helping relationship in favour of dynamic collaboration and client autonomy. There is growing recognition of the client as the 'expert by experience' – that practitioners are not the exclusive holders of expertise. There is an acknowledgement within the mental health professions that the healing skills that are the foundation of their practice are widely disseminated in society among lay helpers. There is an increasing openness about personal vulnerabilities that professional helpers share with the rest of humanity. It is a consciousness of these fundamental issues that can prevent mental health workers from becoming role-bound parodies of the benevolent, authoritative psychiatric professional.

Breggin (1997), in talking about what he calls a *healing presence*, argues that helping has more to do with *being* than doing. It has to do with relating in an empathic and loving way and finding within us the psychological and spiritual resources to nourish and empower the other person. Similarly, Heron (2001) describes a *quality of grace* as the primary source of effective helping. He describes the attributes of this healing presence as:

> *a warm concern for and an acceptance of the other. An openness and attunement to a person's experiential reality. A grasp of what the other needs for their essential flourishing. The ability to facilitate the realisation of those needs in appropriate ways, and the capacity to be with people in an authentic way. (p. 11)*

The person-to-person relationship

The person-centred relationship is more about being than doing. It is a basic philosophy rather than a technique, which involves being with people in a way that creates a climate for growth and change. Rogers, like other humanistic psychologists, believed implicitly in the actualising tendency – a drive towards the constructive expression of our innate potential as cognisant, social, emotional, sexual and spiritual beings. There are times when the realisation of our potential can be blocked, with the result that our self-concept is out of harmony with our core self, and it is this dissonance that creates a great deal of distress and dysfunction.

This process of individuation is of course not passively determined by our psycho-biological heritage but is much more of a dynamic process in which the conscious 'I' engages interpersonally and intrapersonally in the construction of self. In Rogers' view the construction of a valued and authentic self depends on a flow of positive regard from caregivers which affirms an emergent self that is consistent with our core being. If this is lacking in our developmental experience then we become what Rogers referred to as victims of *conditions of worth*. Our capacity to feel positive about ourselves is dependent on us thinking, feeling and behaving in certain ways, ways that others will find worthy of love and respect, but often ways that make authentic living almost impossible. It is a way of being based on the internalised value judgements of others.

Distress experience emerging from the depths of the psyche disrupts the fragile self, an effect compounded by having that experience attributed to psychiatric illness. The self then becomes further undermined by stigmatisation, discrimination and loss of citizenship which so often are the consequence of becoming a psychiatric patient. It is the case that for many the quest in recovery is the quest for personhood. Only through the reconstruction of self, a self that has a sustainable feeling of worth, can people move towards being autonomous adults, living in ways that bring some measure of fulfilment.

Given a nurturing relational experience, our emergent self can move towards being a fully functioning person. This is the challenge of helping relationships in the recovery process. As Rogers puts it:

> *All individuals have within themselves the ability to guide their own lives in a manner that is both personally satisfying and socially constructive. In a particular type of helping relationship, we free the individual to find their inner wisdom and confidence and they will make increasingly healthier and more constructive choices. (Carl Rogers, cited in Kirschenbaum & Henderson 1990, p. xiv)*

It was Rogers' contention, sustained experientially in his practice and supported by research, that six *core conditions* are necessary to facilitate growth and change. These are:

* Psychological contact or engagement
* Incongruence, vulnerability and anxiety of the client
* Authenticity or congruence of the helper
* Warm acceptance or unconditional positive regard of the helper
* Empathic understanding of the client's world which the helper is able to communicate
* Client perceives at least to a minimal degree the helper's authenticity, acceptance and empathy.

While a lot of attention has been paid to the helper's authenticity, acceptance and empathy, there has been less focus given to the client's perception of those attitudes in the helper and the degree of engagement. It is self-evident that however efficacious the core conditions are, they will be of no value if the client is unable or unwilling to engage. Some clients may recoil from the presence of the helper. The expression of these core values may be distrusted, since in the main arena of social life these relational ways of being are often muted, if present at all. Relating in this way may also give rise to some confusion about the nature of the relationship, particularly where person-centred helping is taking place outside of a formal psychotherapeutic space.

Unless a person is able to be receptive and responsive at least to a minimal degree to the helper's presence, then recovery work cannot begin, and there is no doubt that for many people engagement with mental health professionals can be understandably difficult. In a review of engagement with services the Sainsbury Centre for Mental Health (1998) estimates that 15 000 people in Britain with enduring mental health problems are disengaged from services. There are manifold reasons for this including, crucially, a negative experience of statutory services in the past. Many people have been subjected to traumatising experiences of hospital, being compulsory detained, restrained physically, secluded, given medication forcibly or coercively. Campbell (2000), in reflecting on his own admissions and his wish for a 'controlled breakdown', comments that the process *stripped him of power* and was lacking in respect for his integrity. He concludes that it is the compulsory, coercive element in mental health care that goes some way towards 'explaining why many psychiatric patients look back on their time in hospital as a punishment' (p. 59). Little wonder that a legacy of distrust persists and people shy away from statutory mental health services.

While this difficult ethical question of whether an enforced loss of liberty can be fully reconciled with the ethos of care remains, this is not the only important issue in the reluctance to engage. As important is the belief, implicit in a psychiatric referral, that there is something 'mad' or 'ill' about the way a person is experiencing the world and themselves. It may be the cause of suffering, it may be dysfunctional, but many people will resist the notion that it is madness or illness. McGruder (2001) argues that to symptomatise unusual experience may have the effect of 'turning off' conversations that are part of the quest for meaning and identity reconstruction. She advocates respectful listening, without labelling, acknowledging that psychiatry is open to bias and that tempering our enthusiasm for pharmacological interventions 'can go a long way towards establishing ourselves as allies in recovery' (p. 73).

It is therefore vitally important to be able to engage with people in a way that both values and seeks to understand their phenomenological world. Miller (2000) makes a strong case for 'personal consciousness integration' to be incorporated into recovery programmes. She argues that non-ordinary states of consciousness are widely experienced and potentially growth enhancing. They become problematic and may be labelled 'psychotic' when they are externalised, projected and acted out indiscriminately, precipitating a state of confusion and conflict between an individual's inner world and consensual reality. Often unresolved emotional issues are activated in non-ordinary states of consciousness and contribute to an experience of psycho-spiritual overwhelm. The common psychiatric response to this experience is to prescribe increasing doses of neuroleptic drugs which may suppress the manifestation of non-ordinary states of consciousness such as voices, visions and unusual thoughts, but which in doing so deprive people of a potentially growthful experience:

> *Most recipients of psychiatric rehabilitation services cease to discuss their*
> *non ordinary experiences with professionals; they have learned that the*
> *most profound and challenging experiences of their lives are ignored and labelled*
> *as psychopathology by the mental health system. When they express anxiety*
> *about these experiences typically their medication is increased. (Miller 2000,*
> *p. 346)*

Miller argues that personal consciousness integration is an alternative response to 'psychotic' phenomena. In this *educative-consultative growth model* a person's unusual experience becomes the focus of the dialogue with the mental health professionals. An increasingly open discussion about the experience is encouraged in which there is a search for personal meaning and an exploration of the individual's emotional reactions. Unresolved traumas, losses or fears may appear in the dialogue or are present on the edge of the individual's awareness and can be disentangled from the non-ordinary state of consciousness. There is then a basis for the practitioner to offer information about the nature of altered states of consciousness which clients may find normalising and affirming, and to suggest strategies for reducing anxiety about their unusual experiences. Finally, sessions are targeted towards integrating the experience into a newly emerging and valued sense of self. A process such as personal consciousness integration will only occur in the context of a trusting, respectful relationship in which the individual feels supported and has their personal experiences affirmed and normalised.

Over the last few years there has been some interesting person-centred work done with people who find it difficult to make psychological contact (Prouty et al 2002). This contact impairment can be interpersonal or in relation to self. Being with some people who are caught in a continuing dysfunctional state can be like entering an affective void. Words might be exchanged but there is no meeting of hearts and minds and it is as if they are sealed off from others and from themselves. Other people seem so adrift in their altered state of consciousness that anchoring themselves to the reality of another's presence is difficult. A young man I have worked with for several years seems to exemplify this sealed off way of being. It is difficult to move beyond superficial, emotionally neutral conversation and any attempt to engage at a deeper level is met with evasion. His most poignant and revealing communications are through his body language – deep sighs, alarmed looks, displaced tension, moments of distraction, hurriedness, overdressing, all of which speak of anxiety leaking from his sealed off inner world. Beyond all this fearfulness and the psychological sanctuary/prison he has created for himself I have an intuitive image of a warm, funny, artistic, intelligent young man. I think his breakdown cast him into a bleak and paranoid landscape which was so frightening that to risk returning there to learn and grow from that experience is daunting. Yet I feel he will make that journey. To reflect back to him some of his bodily expressions takes us on short excursions into his inner world. It is a beginning!

Genuineness as a way of being

Can we be real and authentic in our helping relationships? Can we cast aside professional or personal façades and be genuinely ourselves in our conversations with people in their quest for personal growth and recovery? Can we be sufficiently aware of the flow of our inner experience – thoughts, images and feelings – in the course of our interactions with others and use such awareness judiciously? Rogers (1978) underlined the significance of genuineness to helping relationships in the following statement: 'The more transparent a helper can be the greater the likelihood the client will change and grow in a constructive manner' (p. 9).

This notion of being congruent is still as much of an anathema to many mental health professionals today as it was 40 years ago when Rogers was developing his interpersonal theory of change. It challenges us to come out from behind the role of the expert, the mystique of the psychotherapeutic stance, the mask of sanity and to be fully present with people in compassionate ways. This is fundamental to recovery, because if we cannot meet with someone person to person, then we cannot help that person in his/her quest for meaning, self-acceptance and self-esteem.

Let us think about why this is and what it means in practice. How is it going to be possible for the client to trust that someone truly believes in them, accepts them with all their faults, failings and weaknesses, has regard for them, values their qualities, strengths and potentials, if they feel that person is being inauthentic in their relationship with them? How can they grow and change, how can they reconfigure their sense of self and reality if they cannot trust that what is reflected back to them is real?

What genuineness means is that we are *dedicated and intentional* in our desire to be as open and fully present as we can be with people (Mearns & Thorne 2000). Being authentic does not mean that we have to disclose everything that we experience, rather that we should be bold enough to share what could be of value to the other person in their quest for growth and change. Thorne (1992), in his biographical appraisal of Rogers' life and work, comments that the value of appropriate self-revelation was given greater impetus and credence as the result of Rogers' work with people suffering from 'psychosis'. Reality can be viewed as a relational phenomenon, in that we test out the validity and meaning of our perceptions, of our self and our world in the social matrix of everyday life. It follows that in troubled states of mind a client will require someone to be more than an accepting, empathic mirror and need to experience the helper's humanity and reality in order to anchor them in a coherent world. Without appropriate sharing, the dialogue loses its vibrant, collaborative, facilitative quality.

Acceptance as a way of being

Many people suffer from such chronically low self-esteem that it predisposes them to depression, anxiety and lack of confidence and this is often a fundamental part of the problem in living for which people seek help through the mental health services. Unfortunately the process of becoming a patient can reinforce that sense of worthlessness and the social impoverishment and stigma that many people with continuing mental health problems encounter can erode self-belief and self-regard still further. Relating to people in warm accepting ways, respecting their humanity and uniqueness, is an antidote to these assaults on an individual's self-esteem. In a powerful heartfelt cry against the oppressive attitudes within the mental health system and in wider society, Wallcroft (2000) underlines the need for warmly accepting attitudes:

> *The experience of many survivors is of being misheard, devalued, written off and damaged because of others' fear of madness. Sharing our stories finally gave us the courage to believe that we are not mad: we are angry that what we are saying is not the result of deluded thinking; distressing things really have happened to us and our distress and anger is often a reasonable and comprehensible response to real life situations that have robbed us of our power and taught us helplessness.*

Low self-esteem has its origins in the formative experiences of early life. We soon learn what is lovable and acceptable and that certain forms of behaviour are prohibited. The child whose playful exuberance is disapproved of may lose touch with their capacity to be enthusiastic, spontaneous and playful. If our distress and comfort seeking behaviour are ignored, we may grow up denying our emotional hurts and needs. We may come to believe that we have no legitimate right to emotional support from others and that come what may we should cope. If we grow up and into adulthood predominantly exposed to a family system, school system, work system and marital system characterised by conditional regard, our sense of self and our self-worth will be vulnerable. In addition contemporary Western society makes it very difficult to sustain self-esteem, bombarded as we are with commercially inspired idealised images of the man or woman we should aspire to be and the life we should aspire to live.

A number of terms have been used to describe acceptance – being non judgemental, prizing, respect, valuing, affirming – all of which communicate an attitude of positive regard. It is not an easy attitude to hold. Accepting some people can be difficult, prejudicial attitudes colour our interaction, feelings of disapproval, irritation or antipathy surface into consciousness or lurk on the edge of our awareness. Where such feelings exist, it is worth challenging ourselves with questions such as: 'Who does this person remind me of?' 'Do the attributes of this person that I find irritating also belong to me?' 'How is it that I become bored/impatient/critical/distant when I am with this person?' Listening openly to ourselves for an answer to these questions can bring into awareness our projections, prejudices and unacknowledged needs and fears. Acceptance as a way of being requires us to be accepting towards ourselves. That means being willing to confront our own vulnerabilities, inadequacies and failings. It means recognising our shadow side and within it the capacity to think, feel and act in ways that are the antithesis of the moral and ethical aspirations and imperatives that govern our lives. It means recognising our common humanity – as Sullivan (1953) famously observed, commenting on his work with people experiencing psychotic phenomena, 'We are all more alike than different'.

An 'us and them' split has characterised the separation, both physically and psychologically, of the mad from the sane throughout the last two centuries in Western society. It serves as a defence against our deepest fear that all too easily reason can be lost and unfettered destructive passions unleashed; a fear that has its origin in the erroneous belief that inside the thin veneer of socially attuned civilised man lurks a barbarian. Such an image has become the stereotype of madness. In Christianised culture we have been impregnated with the doctrine of original sin, with its implication that something bad lurks at the heart of humankind which must be contained and constrained. But could we not argue that the cruel and perverse acts of human beings are distortions of our true nature and that rather than the bearer of original sin, humankind is the bearer of original blessing, that is a capacity for goodness? Despite the persistence of dark images, there are signs that madness is being divested of its historical associations and its sanitised clinical counterpart.

Empathy as a way of being

It is a curious fact that once the assessment and diagnostic process is complete there is a diminishing amount of dialogue between mental health professionals and people seeking to discern the meaning of experiences in the context of their lives. It is as if once defined and categorised according to the practitioner's theoretical model, that is the end of the matter. Talk is then about the frequency and severity of symptoms, the relief and management of those symptoms and little else. While for some people there is relief in a diagnosis of their altered mood or extraordinary state of consciousness as illness, for others this is not an explanation that is acceptable. In a moving personal account of his experience of 'psychosis', John Modrow writes:

> I cannot think of anything more destructive to one's sense of worth as a human being than to believe that the inner core of one's being is sick – that one's thoughts, values, feelings and beliefs are merely the meaningless symptoms of a sick mind. (Cited in McGruder 2001, p. 66)

For many people their greatest need is to make sense of what is happening to them, to find some meaning for this perplexing, disturbing, overwhelming experience in the context of their lives. It is only when some shared understanding has been arrived at that they can reconfigure who they are and move on in their lives. Mental health workers can help in this quest for meaning if they are able to be an *empathic companion*: someone willing to listen, to enter the world of the client's lived experience and communicate to the individual what they sense of that world as accurately as possible. Rogers, in his evocative style, put it this way: empathy

> involves being sensitive, moment to moment, to the changing felt meanings that flow in the other person, to the fear or rage or sadness or confusion or whatever she/he is experiencing. It means temporarily living in his/her life, moving about in it delicately without making judgements, sensing meaning of which he/she is scarcely aware, but not trying to uncover feelings of which the person is unaware as that would be too threatening. It includes communicating your sensing of his/her world as you look with fresh and unfrightened eyes at elements of which the individual is fearful. It means frequently checking with him/her the accuracy of your sensing and being guided by the responses you receive. You are a confident companion to the person in his/her inner world. (1980, p. 142)

There is an important 'as if' quality about empathy – it is 'as if' we are entering someone else's world, trying to see it through their eyes, but never losing touch with our own reality. Even so it is not uncommon to take on and take away the feelings we find there, or conversely project our own feelings and meanings on to the other's personal world, particularly if that person's emotional struggles and problems of living resonate with our own. As with the other core conditions, empathy is a way of being and relating that we cultivate and value in our personal lives and extend to ourselves. Breggin (1997) argues that *empathic self-transformation* is at the heart of being a healing presence for others – we need to know our own emotional landscape if we are to become confident companions to others in their emotional turmoil. If we can face our own emotional pain, come through and be strengthened by it, then we are less likely to be reduced to fearful helplessness by the distress of others and will be able to deal with crises with compassionate calm.

The concept of the wounded healer has impinged itself on the consciousness of the mental health professions over the past decade. During that time many mental health workers, some quoted in this book, have courageously 'come out' and openly written and spoken about their own vulnerabilities. Many people who have struggled with overwhelming distress and despair have 'come through' to become the articulate and empathically representative voices of the service user movement. I do not think it is overstating the case to say that the challenge of the survivor/consumer movement to psychiatry and the mental health system has sown the seed of change in professional attitudes and practice and influenced the reconfiguration of mental health services in Britain. Others have brought their ability to relate in deeply empathic ways to advocacy or volunteer work in the mental health field. The idea that the gift of healing is a corollary of woundedness has a long history. In non-technological societies healers and shamans are usually people who have travelled in the outer reaches of the human psyche, to the psycho-spiritual realm, where both disorder and disease and harmony and healing have their origins. They have returned with knowledge of practices – herbalistic or ritualistic or spiritualistic – that release the intrinsic healing process in the sufferer. Perhaps it is not stretching the point too far to say that modern psychotherapeutic practitioners who have suffered their own psycho-spiritual wounds and have recovered through a 'pilgrimage within' are inheritors of the shamanistic tradition. They, more than any mental health worker, can draw deeply on their experiential knowledge and be empathically aware companions in others' journeys of recovery.

Empathy is a multifaceted quality in relationships. It gently follows and leads people in a process of knowing themselves more deeply. It attunes us to the emotional dimension of a person's experience, which is often to be found on the edge of awareness, and can facilitate the acknowledgement and discharge of feeling. It acts as a guide to the times when it can be helpful to share knowledge, knowledge that is existentially relevant to the person seeking help (Heron 2001). The experience of empathic understanding is immensely supportive, as captured here by Rogers (1980) in a personal reflection:

> *I like being heard. A number of times in my life I have felt myself bursting with insoluble problems, or going round and round in tormented circles, during one period being overcome by feelings of worthlessness and despair. I think I have been more fortunate than most in finding at these times, individuals who have been able to hear me and thus rescue me from the chaos of my feelings, individuals who have been able to hear my meanings a little more deeply than I have known them. These persons have heard me without judging me, diagnosing me or evaluating me. They have just listened and clarified and responded to me at all the levels at which I was communicating. I can testify that when you are in psychological distress and someone really hears you without passing judgement on you, without trying to take responsibility for you, without trying to mould you it feels damn good! At these times it has relaxed the tension, the despair, the confusions that have been part of the experience. When I have been listened to and have been heard, I am able to perceive my world in a new way and go on. It is astonishing how elements that seemed insoluble become soluble when someone listens, how confusions that seemed irredeemable turn into relatively clear flowing streams when one is heard. I have deeply appreciated the times I have experienced this sensitive, empathic, concentrated listening and being heard. (p. 12)*

An intuitive way of being

In a fascinating study of intuition in psychotherapeutic practice Rachel Charles describes how the ascendancy of logic and reason has left intuition in a subordinate position to the extent that it has been largely disregarded by psychologists and psychotherapists. This seems extraordinary, given that intuition 'can be pivotal in understanding human dilemmas and in helping solve life's problems' (Charles 2004).

The mental health professions, in pursuit of professional credibility in an age of evidence-based practice, have largely turned their backs on intuitive care. Reflecting on my own work I recollect many occasions when I now wish I had trusted my intuition rather than cognitive appraisal as a basis for my response. I recall with lingering sadness and regret a talented man who hanged himself on a local heath, having spoken with me at length two days before. I knew subjectively that all was not well, but by all objective criteria he appeared to be progressing in his recovery from a severe depression. There was a mild euphoric sense to his manner that I interpreted as the joy of having come through, but which I see now as the gladness of a mind resolved to seek the ultimate end to his suffering.

What is it that creates within us this state of knowingness that seems to arrive unheralded and complete in our consciousness? The experience of not knowing how we know, we just know! Intuition is not the same as empathy although they are related attributes. Empathy is an attunement to the experience of another person, often although not exclusively at an emotional level. There is an element of resonance with the other person's experience and we get a palpable impression of what that lived experience is like. Empathic attunement is a vital element in social cohesion – we could not relate to each other with consideration and compassion were it not for our capacity to transpose ourselves into another's world. It is a facet of human relating that allows us to feel deeply connected to each other and is an antidote to alienation. Often empathic understanding has to be consciously worked at. We seek to understand an experience and its meaning through a reflective conversation, gradually finding our way into another's lived experience. At its deepest level it feels like a merging of one's consciousness with that of another, yet never losing that sense of separateness.

By comparison, intuition seems to appear in our minds in the form of connections, thoughts, feelings, images or felt senses which are not the product of any conscious rational process. It is therefore not surprising that throughout history the intuitive self has been linked to paranormal phenomena. In ancient Greek civilisation intuitive insight or understanding was often attributed to daemons or gods. Famously Socrates relied on a personal daemon for guidance in times of duress, a phenomenon played out fictionally to the full in Philip Pullman's trilogy *His Dark Materials*, in which the central character, Lyra, has a guardian daemon. Carl Jung, whose life and work was richly intuitive, spoke of a Philemon – a winged creature that was a harbinger of insights from the unconscious realms of his psyche. Other great thinkers have equated intuition with the spiritual or transpersonal dimension of their lives. Mystical experiences whether religious or secular can be intense life-changing occurrences, *ultimate* or *peak* experiences within which we witness revelations of truth, beauty and love, often accompanied by a sense of the divine nature of all things. When I was in my early forties and going through a period tormented by depressive thoughts, sleepless in the dead of night I heard a voice saying, 'All will be well'. It was the nature of the voice, an embodiment of love and compassion, that left me at once relieved beyond measure. I have not heard the voice since, but echoes of it remain and it has left a measure of stillness in my psyche that has enabled me to hold on to my sanity in the face of life's adversities.

Many poets, writers and artists depend on intuitive experience for their inspiration and creative flow. In a sense the poem writes itself and the painting paints itself. Works of art are not consciously rational processes: the act of creation comes predominantly from the imaginative, intuitive realms of the brain.

Intuition has a valid place in the care process. We should not be shy of drawing on images, feelings, words, phrases, ideas and felt senses that surface unbidden in our consciousness in relation to people we are working with. Such intuition can provide helpful insights into a person's distress and problems in living. It can guide the flow and substance of the interaction and, used judiciously, can help deepen the relationship. Intuition seems to be a subliminal response to non-verbal cues, to the said and the unsaid, to the context of a person's life. It stirs our imagination and memory. It reverberates in our unconscious and offers up its wisdom. Sometimes we need to allow ourselves to be confused, to be content not to know what to say or do. If we wait expectantly, a way forward will usually emerge from the creative unconscious. Of course our intuition can be wrong and it is easy to overstate the case for the superiority of its insights and solutions. It seems wise to subject our intuitive inclinations to cognitive scrutiny, to check out the validity and appropriateness of our understanding and proposed actions. But being alive to our intuitive powers, cultivating them, can lead to a more creative way of being and relating.

Not only should we be alive to this intuitive function within ourselves but we should seek to cultivate it in the people who seek our help on their recovery journeys. Many people recognise that still small voice inside which, if we would only listen to it, acts as a guide in life choices. Over the past few years I have worked with a gifted young man recovering from what one might describe as extraordinary, sometimes overwhelming, states of consciousness that have had a disruptive impact on his life. A significant part of the healing process for him has been to intuitively seek an inner source of wisdom for an understanding of his perplexing experiences and as a guide to his recovery. The source has become personified in his mind as a beneficent entity that he is able to contact at will through automatic writing. Reading some of this remarkable script I have been struck by the loving kindness, insightfulness and pragmatism of this inner voice – a voice that he has now come to trust and value. I suspect this phenomenon is a manifestation of the archetype of great wisdom and of great love that resides in us all and his breakdown has enabled him to receive a great gift that could be an inspiring and sustaining facet of his life.

So how do we begin to develop our intuition? Firstly we need to challenge the prevailing belief that intuition is anathema to the rational mind. We should not mystify it, but recognise it for what it is: a coalescence of impressions, thoughts, images, feelings and felt senses, mostly perceived subliminally, stirred in our imagination and memory and synthesised into a meaningful whole, in which form it reaches consciousness. It is a valid source of knowledge about ourselves and our world and is the wellspring of creative living. We must free ourselves from the dogma that abounds in psychiatry to create sufficient space for intuition to flourish. If we cling to an established view we are unlikely to be open to intuitive insights which challenge an 'existing truth'. Although it takes courage in the scientifically orientated culture of psychiatric medicine, I believe we should bring more of our intuitive self into client work, clinical reviews and supervision. Often when I meet with clients, we will start with a five minute meditation. I find that this helps clear the mind, allows us to become more attuned to each other and to be open to any intuitive thoughts, feelings, images that present themselves to be worked with.

There probably are, as Rowan (1993) suggests, different levels of intuitive functioning which depend on the level of our psycho-spiritual development. The more we can accept and be open to *the fullness of our self*, the more autonomous we are able to be in our thinking, the more regular and dependable this facet of our mental functioning becomes. As our intuitive life becomes richer, it expresses itself not only in thoughts but in images too. These metaphors and symbols from the unconscious are postcards from the outer reaches, from the archetypal realms of human experience. According to Jung, archetypes are the deepest patterns of psychic functioning, the imprints of humankind's history. They are the stuff of mythology, the roots of the soul, and they evoke feelings, images and themes that are universal. To be open to this inheritance brings us back to a realisation of our history and nature and frees us from the superficial preoccupations of everyday life. Having been professionally educated to value logical, analytic understanding, intuitive knowing has been a distrusted faculty. Yet it has remained a strong presence in my work and personal life and in recent years I have learned to draw with more confidence on this universal, yet neglected, source of wisdom.

Becoming a person-centred helper

Being a person-centred helper is not straightforward. The qualities of genuineness, acceptance, empathy and intuitiveness we aspire to and seek to communicate in our relationships are deceptively difficult to develop and sustain. It is no easy thing to be with people in their distress and despair as they struggle with the challenges and adversities of being human and offer them 'acceptance where there has been rejection, understanding where there has been indifference and mutuality where there has been an abuse of power' (Thorne 1998). Person-centredness is often challenged for its 'naivety' and its misplaced trust in the human spirit. The core conditions are often seen by the psychiatric professions as simply a necessary backdrop against which 'real' helping takes place. Sometimes the needs and expectations of people seeking help seem too great, their fragility too perilous, their confusion unfathomable, their behaviour irredeemable. Despite all this the person-centred approach seems to me to offer the most cogent philosophy on which to base recovery relationships. If we see the essence of recovery as a process of growth and development, or as a spiritual awakening, or as a process of social inclusion or, less prosaically, simply as getting on with life, then this is most likely to occur in the context of empowering relationships.

Most professional education does not in my experience create a learning milieu in which the core conditions can develop. For person-centredness to become

149

internalised as a philosophy and way of being, it needs to permeate the whole learning culture and the organisational culture of mental health services. This means that learning would be student-centred with relationships between students and lecturers more egalitarian. A student-centred, adult-orientated approach to teaching helpfully mirrors the kind of collaborative relationship student practitioners would seek to establish with clients. There would be respect for experiential knowledge. Students would become resourceful learners with much more freedom to determine how they learn. In other words the prevailing culture would be one of empowerment, not one where fear and dependency were the evident characteristics. Within the context of student-centred culture it would be possible to introduce structures to explore experientially relationship skills and emotional competence. Emotional competence means that helping is less likely to be contaminated by the emotional legacies of the helper's past hurts (Heron 2001). Heron's view, borne out in my experience, is that there is a lot of 'contaminated helping' taking place, both by lay and professional mental health workers. The history of psychiatry is littered with examples of the abuse of power – physical, coercive, oppressive – representing the shadow side of helping relationships (Watkins 2001).

Central to person-centred helping is the practitioner's commitment to self-awareness and personal development. The working environment should provide a culture in which the 'personal in the professional' can be acknowledged and examined as a necessary part of the quest for excellence in practice. Traditionally a rather macho ethos has permeated the culture of psychiatric services. A high value has been placed on emotional containment, cognitive knowing and tough mindedness in the face of the demands and vicissitudes of working life. To be out of step with that conception of the 'ideal psychiatric practitioner' is to risk being thought professionally inadequate. But how can we carry the emotional burden of the work and not become burnt out, indifferent and cynical, if we cannot reflect openly on the complex emotional issues raised by the work? It can be difficult to accept the dependency needs of a client to be cared for and looked after – until that need has less primacy and can be met through the mutuality of adult–adult relationships – if we do not acknowledge our own dependency needs. It can be difficult to accept non-compliance if we do not recognise our need for control and the anxieties that surface when that control is lost. We may not recognise a client's emotional cues or respond appropriately to their distress if we cannot face and deal with our own emotional pain. These kinds of scenarios in the art of helping seem to me unequivocally to make the case for a working culture where support and supervision are given high priority and where personal development work is recognised as a legitimate facet of professional education.

The team – the recovery team, the crisis and home treatment team, the outreach team – has a big role to play in sustaining the energy, commitment and creativity of its individual members. Any system will go through periods of dysfunction where it is no longer so effective in meeting the needs of members or fulfilling its functions. The symptoms of that dysfunction are that practitioners split off and operate in a more isolated way; divisions and divisiveness appear between members; team protocols are disregarded; discord flows under the surface and leaks out in resentment and angry disputes; commitment to the team and the work diminishes; cynicism creeps in and begins to have a corrosive effect on the aspirations of the service.

In dysfunctional teams, individuals feel powerless and oppressed, no longer feeling heard, valued or supported. Ultimately, unless these issues can be openly addressed and resolved and the cohesiveness of the team restored, the quality of the work suffers and the sickness and attrition rate will increase. Maintaining the wellbeing, cohesiveness and efficiency of the staff team can be mediated through structures that allow the team to meet regularly in a safe space, where the agenda is concerned with addressing the emotional life of the team, including the shadow side of the staff group and the wider psychiatric system in which it operates.

We are all part of an ever widening system by which we are influenced and upon which, in turn, we have an influence. One can think of the family, the neighbourhood, the town, the country, the international community and the natural world as social and ecological systems by which we are sustained. We, collectively and individually, have a responsibility to act within these systems to contribute wherever and however we can to healing the body and soul of humanity and this world that we occupy for such a short span of time. Recovery then is a universal quest, and is, if we are to survive, the most important quest that humankind faces as the 21st century unfolds.

Addendum

Wild geese

You do not have to be good.
You do not have to walk on your knees
for a hundred miles through the desert, repenting.
You only have to let the soft animal of your body
  love what it loves.
Tell me about despair, yours, and I will tell you mine.
Meanwhile the world goes on.
Meanwhile the sun and the clear pebbles of the rain
are moving across the landscapes,
over the prairies and deep trees,
the mountains and the rivers.
Meanwhile the wild geese, high in the clean blue air
are heading home again.
Whoever you are, no matter how lonely,
the world offers itself to your imagination,
calls to you like the wild geese, harsh and exciting –
over and over announcing your place
in the family of things.

Mary Oliver

(Reproduced from Oliver, M 2006 Dream Work. Grove/Atlantic, Inc., New York, with kind permission of the publishers)

References

Aderhold V, Gottwalz E 2004 Family therapy in schizophrenia: replacing ideology with openness. In: Read J, Mosher L, Bentall R (eds) Models of madness. Brunner-Routledge, Hove, East Sussex

Ahern L, Fisher D 2001 Recovery at your own pace. Journal of Psychosocial Nursing and Mental Health Services 39:4

Ainsworth M 1991 Attachments and other affectional bonds across the life cycle. In: Parks C, Stevenson-Hinde J, Marris P (eds) Attachment across the life cycle. Tavistock/Routledge, London

Allen J J, Schager R, Hitt S 1998 The efficacy of acupuncture in the treatment of major depression in women. Psychological Science 9(5):397–401

Anthony W 1993 Recovery from mental illness: the guiding vision of the mental health service system in the 1990s. Psychosocial Rehabilitation Journal 16(4):11–23

Astley N (ed) 2002 Staying alive: real poems for unreal times. Bloodaxe, Tarset, Northumberland

Baker S 2000 Environmentally friendly? Patients' views of conditions on psychiatric wards. Mind, London

Barker P, Buchanan Barker P 2004 Spirituality and mental health. Whurr, London

Barker P, Campbell P, Davidson C (eds) 1999 From the ashes of experience: reflections on madness, survival and growth. Whurr, London

Barry K L, Zeber J E, Blow F C et al 2003 Effect of Strengths model versus assertive community treatment of participant outcomes and utilization: two year follow up. Psychiatric Rehabilitation Journal 26(3):268–277

Barton R 1976 Institutional neurosis. Wright, London

Bebbington P, Kuipers E 1994 The predictive utility of expressed emotion in schizophrenia: an aggregate analysis. Psychological Medicine 21:707–718.

Bentall R 2003 Madness explained: psychosis and human nature. Penguin Books, London

Berry T 1999 The collected thoughts of Thomas Berry. Audio programme. Center for the Study of the Universe, Mill Valley, CA

Bhugra D, Bahl V (eds) 1999 Ethnicity: an agenda for mental health. Gaskell, London

Bindman J, Tighe J, Thornicroft G et al 2002 Poverty, social services and compulsory psychiatric admission in England. Social Psychiatry and Psychiatric Epidemiology 37:340–345

Birchwood M, Todd P, Jackson C 1998 Early intervention in psychosis: the critical period hypothesis. British Journal of Psychiatry 172(Suppl. 33):53–59

Birchwood M, Iqbal Z, Chadwick P et al 2000 Cognitive approach to depression and suicidal thinking in psychosis 1: ontogeny of post psychotic depression. British Journal of Psychiatry 177:516–521

Bly R 1990 Iron John. Element Books, Longmead, Dorset

Bowlby J 1988 A secure base: clinical applications of attachment theory. Tavistock/Routledge, London

Bracken P, Thomas P 2001 Post-psychiatry: a new direction for mental health. British Medical Journal 322:724–727

Brazier D (ed) 1993 Beyond Carl Rogers. Constable, London

Breggin P 1993 Toxic psychiatry. Harper Collins, London

Breggin P 1996 Spearheading a transformation. In: Breggin P, Stern E M (eds) Psychosocial approaches to deeply disturbed people. Haworth Press, New York

Breggin P 1997 The heart of being helpful: empathy and the creation of healing presence. Springer, New York

British Psychological Society Report June 2000 Recent advances in the understanding of mental illness and psychotic experiences. British Psychological Society, Leicester

Butzlaff R L, Hooley J M 1999 Expressed emotion and psychiatric relapse: a meta analysis. Archives of General Psychiatry 55:547–552

Byng-Hall J 1995 Rewriting family scripts. Guilford Press, New York

Campbell J 1993 The hero with a thousand faces. Fontana Press, London

Campbell J 2004 Pathways to bliss. New World Library, Novato, California

Campbell P 2000 Challenging loss of power. In: Read J, Reynolds J (eds) Speaking our minds. Palgrave Macmillan, Basingstoke

Camus A 1955 The myth of Sisyphus. Penguin Books, London

Caplan C 1964 Principles of preventative psychiatry. Tavistock, London

Chadwick P 1997 Schizophrenia, the positive perspective. In search of dignity for schizophrenic people. Routledge, London

Chadwick P, Birchwood M, Trower P 1996 Cognitive therapy for delusions, voices and paranoia. John Wiley, Chichester

Chamberlin J 1999 Confessions of a non-compliant patient. National Empowerment Centre newsletter article. Available online. http://www.power2u.org/articles/recovery/confessions.html (accessed 28 August 2006)

Chamberlin J 2004 User-run services. In: Read J, Moscher L, Bentall R (eds) Models of madness: psychological, social and biological approaches to schizophrenia. Brunner-Routledge, Hove, Sussex

Champ S 1999 A most precious thread. In: Barker P, Campbell P, Davidson C (eds) From the ashes of experience: reflections on madness survival and growth. Whurr, London

Charles R 2004 Intuition in psychotherapy and counselling. Whurr, London

Ciompi L 1980 The natural history of schizophrenia in the long term. British Journal of Psychiatry 136:413–420

Ciompi L 1997 The Soteria concept: theoretical bases and practical 13-year experience with a milieu-therapy approach to acute schizophrenia. Psychiatria et Neurologia Japonica 9:634–650

Coleman R 1999 Recovery an alien concept. Handsell, Gloucester

Conroy C 1999 Fire and ice. In: Barker P, Campbell P, Davidson B (eds) From the ashes of experience. Whurr, London

Crawford T A, Lipsedge M 2004 Seeking help for psychological distress: the interface of Zulu traditional healing and Western biomedicine. Mental Health, Religion and Culture 7(2):131–148

Davidson L 2003 Living outside mental illness: qualitative studies of recovery in schizophrenia. New York University Press, New York

Deegan P E 1988 Recovery: a lived experience of rehabilitation. Psychosocial Rehabilitation Journal 11(4):11–19

Deegan P E 1992 The independent living movement and people with psychiatric disabilities: taking back control over our own lives. Psychosocial Rehabilitation Journal 15(3):3–19

Deegan P E 1993 Recovering a sense of value after being labelled. Journal of Psychosocial Nursing 31(4):7–11

Deegan P E 1997 Recovery and empowerment for people with psychiatric disabilities. Social Work and Health Care 25(3):11–24

Deegan P 1999 Reclaiming your power during medication appointments with your psychiatrist. National Empowerment Centre. Newsletter Article. Available online. http://www.power2u.org/selfhelp/reclaim.html (accessed 27 August 2006)

Demling J, Muller J, Zeller K 2004 High dose St John's wort extract as a daily single dose in the treatment of depression. Nervenheilkunde: Zeitschrift fur Interdisziplinaere Fortbildung 23(3):160–164

Department of Health 1999 National service framework for mental health. HMSO, London

Department of Health 2000 The NHS plan: a plan for investment, a plan for reform. HMSO, London

Department of Health 2001 The journey of recovery: the government's vision for mental health care. Department of Health, London

Department of Health 2002a Women's mental health: into the mainstream. Department of Health, London

Department of Health 2002b Developing services for carers and families of people with mental illness. Department of Health, London

Egan G 2002 The skilled helper. Brooks Cole, Pacific Grove

Falloon I R 1992 Early intervention for first episodes of schizophrenia: a preliminary exploration. Psychiatry 55(1):4–15

Falloon I, Coverdale J, Tannis M et al 1998 Early intervention for schizophrenic disorders: implementing optimal treatment strategies in routine clinical services. British Journal of Psychiatry Supplement 172(33):33–38

Fava G, Rafanelli C, Cazzaro M et al 1998 Well being therapy: a novel approach for residual symptoms of affective disorder. Psychological Medicine 28:475–480

Fava M, Alpert J, Nierenberg A et al 2005 Double blind randomised controlled trial of St John's wort, fluoxetine and placebo in major depressive disorder. Journal of Clinical Psychopharmacology 25(5):441–447

Fernando S 1995 Social realities and mental health. In: Fernando S (ed) Mental health in a multi ethnic society. Routledge, London

Fisher D 1999 Hope, humanity and voice in recovery from mental illness. In: Baker P et al (eds) From the ashes of experience. Whurr, London

Fisher D, Deegan P 1999 Final report of research on recovery from mental illness. National Empowerment Centre, Lawrence, MA

Foner J 1996 Surviving the 'mental health' system with co-counselling. In: Breggin P, Stern E M (eds) Psychosocial approaches to deeply disturbed persons. Haworth Press, New York

Foucault M 1961 Madness and civilization. Routledge, London

Fox M 2002 Creativity: where the divine and the human meet. Jeremy P Tarcher/Penguin, New York

Frankl V (ed) 2004 Man's search for meaning. Rider, London

Fromm E 1976 To have or to be. Abacus, London

Garety P, Fowler D, Kuipers E 2000 Cognitive behavioural therapy for medication resistant symptoms. Schizophrenia Bulletin 26(1):73–86

Geddes J, Freemantle N, Harrison P et al 2000 Atypical antipsychotics in the treatment of schizophrenia. British Medical Journal 321:1371–1376

Gergen K 1990 Therapeutic professionals and the diffusion of deficit. Journal of Mind and Behaviour 11:353–368

Gleeson J, Larson T, McGorry P 2003 Psychological treatment in pre and early psychosis. Journal of the American Academy of Psychoanalysis 31:229–245

Goodman L A, Rosenberg S D, Mueser K T et al 1997 Physical and sexual assault history in women with serious mental illness: prevalence, correlates, treatment and future research directions. Schizophrenia Bulletin 23:685–696

Gray P 2006 The madness of our lives. Jessica Kingsley, London

Grayley-Wetherell R, Morgan S 2001 Active outreach: an independent user evaluation of a model of assertive outreach practice. Sainsbury Centre for Mental Health, London

Greasley P, Chiu L F, Gartland M 2001 The concept of spiritual care in mental health nursing. Journal of Advanced Nursing 33(5):629–637

Hambrook C 2000 Healing through creativity. In: Read J, Reynolds J (eds) Speaking our minds. Palgrave Macmillan, Basingstoke

Harding C M, Brooks G W, Asolaga T et al 1987 The Vermont longitudinal study of persons with severe mental illness. American Journal of Psychiatry 144:718–726

Hardy A 1979 The spiritual nature of man. Clarendon Press, Oxford

Harrison G, Hopper K, Craig T et al 2001 Recovery from psychotic illness. British Journal of Psychiatry 178:506–517

Harrop C, Trower P 2001 Why does schizophrenia develop in late adolescence? Clinical Psychology Review 21:241–265

Heron J 2001 Helping the client. Sage Publications, London

Hill D 1986 Tardive dyskinesia: a worldwide epidemic of irreversible brain damage. In: Eisenberg N, Glasgow D (eds) Current issues in clinical psychology. Gower, Aldershot

Hillman J 1976 Re-visioning psychology. HarperPerennial, New York

Hirst I S 2003 Perspectives of mindfulness. Journal of Psychiatric and Mental Health Nursing 10:359–366

Holden M 2005 Opening to direct revelation. Interfaith Seminary, London

Housden R 2003 Ten poems to change your life. Hodder and Stoughton, London

Hubble M A, Duncan B L, Miller S 1999 The heart and soul of change: what works in therapy. American Psychological Association, Washington DC

Inglesby E 2004 Pilgrimage. In: Barker P, Buchanan-Barker P (eds) Spirituality and mental health. Whurr, London

Jablensky A, Sartorius N, Ernbers G et al 1992 Schizophrenia: manifestations, incidence and course in different cultures. Psychological Medicine. Monograph Supplement 20:1–97

Jamison K Redfield 1993 Touched with fire. Simon and Shuster, New York

Johannessen O 2004 The development of early intervention services. In: Read J, Mosher L, Bentall R (eds) Models of madness. Brunner-Routledge, Hove, East Sussex

Johnson L 2000 Uses and abuses of psychiatry, 2nd edn. Brunner-Routledge, Hove, East Sussex

Kaufmann W (trans and ed), Buber M 1970 I and thou. T & T Clark, Edinburgh

Kemp R, Kirov G, Everitt B et al 1998 Randomised controlled trial of compliance therapy: 18 month follow up. British Journal of Psychiatry 171:319–327

Kinderman P, Cooke A 2000 Recent advances in understanding mental illness and psychotic illness. British Psychological Society, Leicester

Kirschenbaum H, Henderson V (eds) 1990 The Carl Rogers reader. Constable, London

Kuipers E, Leff J, Lam D 2002 Family work in schizophrenia: a practical guide, 2nd edn. Royal College of Psychiatrists, London

LaFond V 2002 Grieving mental illness: a guide for patients and their caregivers, 2nd edn. University of Toronto Press, Toronto

Liberman R P, Kopelowicz A, Ventura J et al 2002 Operational criteria and factors related to recovery from schizophrenia. International Review of Psychiatry 14:256–272

Llorca P M, Chereau I, Bayle F J et al 2002 Tardive dyskinesia and antipsychotics. European Psychiatry 17:129–138

Mabey R 2005 Nature cure. Chatto and Windus, London

McGowry P, Yung A, Francey S et al 2002 Randomized controlled trial of interventions designed to reduce the risk of progression to first episode psychosis in a clinical sample with sub-threshold symptoms. Archives of General Psychiatry 59:921–928

McGruder J 2001 Life experience is not a disease, or, Why medicalising madness is counterproductive to recovery. In: Brown C (ed) Recovery and wellness: models of hope and empowerment for people with mental illness. Haworth Press, New York

Macmin L, Foskett J 2004 Don't be afraid to tell: the spiritual and religious experience of mental health service users in Somerset. Mental Health Religion and Culture 7(1):23–40

Marcelis M, Navarro-Mateu F, Murray R, Selten J P, Van Os J 1998 Urbanization and psychosis: a study of 1942–1978 birth cohorts in the Netherlands. Psychological Medicine 28:871–879

Massey A, Butcher G, Benzies C 2005 Recovery for carers. Meriden 2:4. Available online. http://www.meridenfamilyprogramme.com [In-house magazine of the West Midlands Family Programme]

Mearns D, Thorne B 2000 Person centred therapy today. Sage, London

Mental Health Act Commission 2005 Count me in report. Mental Health Act Commission, London

Mental Health Foundation 1997 Knowing our own minds. Mental Health Foundation, London

Mental Health Foundation 1999 The courage to bare our souls. Mental Health Foundation, London

Mental Health Foundation 2000 Strategies for living. Mental Health Foundation, London

Mental Health Foundation 2002 Taken seriously: the Somerset spirituality project. Mental Health Foundation, London

Miller J 2000 Personal consciousness integration: the next phase of recovery. Psychiatric and Rehabilitation Journal 23(4):342–352

Moore T 1994 Care of the soul. Harper Perennial, New York

Morgan S 2004 Strengths-based practice. Openmind 126(March/April)

Morrison A, Frame L, Larkin W 2003 Relationship between trauma and psychosis: a review and integration. British Journal of Psychology 42:331–353

Mortensen P, Juel K 1993 Mortality and the causes of death in first admitted schizophrenic patients. British Journal of Psychiatry 163:183–189

Mosher L 1999 Soteria and other alternatives to acute psychiatric hospitalisation. Journal of Nervous and Mental Diseases 187:142–149

Mosher L 2003 Two alternative viewpoints: psychotropic drugs and crises. Available online. http://www.moshersoteria.com (accessed 3 October 2003)

Mosher L 2004 Non hospital, non drug intervention with first episode psychosis. In: Read J, Mosher L, Bentall R (eds) Models of madness. Brunner-Routledge, Hove, East Sussex

Mueser K T, Goodman L B, Trumbetta S L et al 1998 Trauma and posttraumatic stress disorder in severe mental illness. Journal of Consulting and Clinical Psychology 66:493–499

Mullen A, Murray L, Happell B 2002 Multiple family group interventions in first episode psychosis: enhancing knowledge and understanding. International Journal of Mental Health Nursing 11:225–232

National Institute for Health and Clinical Excellence 2002 Schizophrenia: core interventions and management of schizophrenia in primary and secondary care. NICE, London

National Institute for Mental Health in England (2005) NIMHE Guiding Statement on Recovery. Available online. http://www.nimhe.csip.org.uk/home (accessed 4 September 2006)

Office of National Statistics 2000a Lifetime experience of stressful life events by type of event and gender: a study of psychiatric morbidity. Office of National Statistics, London

Office of National Statistics 2000b Labour force survey 1998–99. Office of National Statistics, London

O'Haver Day P, Horton Deutsch S 2004 Using mindfulness based therapeutic interventions in psychiatric nursing practice. Part 1: Description and empirical support for mindfulness based interventions. Archives of Psychiatric Nursing 18(5):164–169

O'Toole M, Ohlsen R, Taylor T et al 2004 Treating first episode psychosis: the service user's perspective. A focus group evaluation. Journal of Psychiatric and Mental Health Nursing 11:319–326

Parker U 1999 Talk and tears replaced psychiatric drugs. In: The courage to bare our souls. Mental Health Foundation, London

Pedersen C B, Mortensen P B 2001 Evidence of a dose–response relationship between urbanicity during upbringing and schizophrenia risk. Archives of General Psychiatry 58:1039–1046

Pennings M, Romme M 1998 Hearing voices in patients and non patients. In: Romme M (ed) Understanding voices. Handsell Publishing, Runcorn

Podvoll E 2003 Recovering sanity. a compassionate approach to understanding and treating psychosis. Shambhala Publications, Boston

Power N, Elkins K, Adlard S et al 1998 Analysis of the initial treatment phase in first episode psychosis. British Journal of Psychiatry Supplement 172(33):71–76

Priest P 2006 Walking testimonies. Resurgence 234:26–27

Prouty G, Van Werde D, Portner M 2002 Pre therapy: reaching contact impaired clients. PCCS Books, Ross on Wye

Rapp C A 1998 The strengths model: case management with people suffering from severe and persistent mental illness. Oxford University Press, New York

Read J 2004 Poverty, ethnicity and gender. In: Read J, Mosher L, Bentall R (eds) Models of madness. Brunner-Routledge, Hove, East Sussex

Read J, Haslam N 2004 Public opinion: bad things happen and can drive you crazy. In: Read J, Mosher L, Bentall R (eds) Models of madness. Brunner-Routledge, Hove, East Sussex

Read J, Reynolds J 2000 Speaking our minds: an anthology. Palgrave Macmillan, Basingstoke

Read J, Seymore F, Mosher L 2004 Unhappy families. In: Read J, Mosher L, Bentall R (eds) Models of madness. Brunner-Routledge, Hove, East Sussex

Rector N, Beck A 2002 A clinical review of cognitive therapy for schizophrenia. Current Psychiatry Reports 4:284–292

Reilly D 2005 The evidence for homeopathy. Glasgow Royal Homeopathic Hospital. Available online. http://www.adhom.com/ (accessed 27 August 2006)

Repper J, Perkins R 2003 Social inclusion and recovery: a model for mental health practice. Baillière Tindall, Edinburgh

Roberts G, Wolfson P 2004 The rediscovery of recovery: open to all. Advances in Psychiatric Treatment 10:37–49

Roe D, Chopra M, Wagner B et al 2004 The emerging self in conceptualization and treating mental illness. Journal of Psychosocial Nursing and Mental Health Services 42(2):32–40

Rogers C 1961 On becoming a person. Houghton Mifflin, Boston

Rogers C 1978 Carl Rogers on personal power: inner strength and its revolutionary impact. Constable, London

Rogers C 1980 A way of being. Houghton Mifflin, Boston

Romme M, Escher S 1989 Hearing voices. Schizophrenia Bulletin 15(2):209–216

Romme M, Escher S 1993 Accepting voices. Mind Publications, London

Romme M, Escher S 2000 Making sense of voices. Mind, London

Roschke J, Wolfe C, Muller M et al 2000 The benefit from whole body acupuncture in major depression. Journal of Affective Disorders 57(1–3):73–81

Ross C, Read J 2004 Antipsychotic medication: myths and facts. In: Read J, Mosher L, Bentall R (eds) Models of madness. Brunner-Routledge, Hove, East Sussex

Roszak T, Gomes M, Kanner A (eds) 1995 Ecopsychology: restoring the earth, healing the mind. Sierra Club Books, San Franciso

Rowan J 1993 The transpersonal self: psychotherapy and counselling. Routledge, London

Rushing W, Ortega S 1979 Socioeconomic status and mental disorder. American Journal of Sociology 84:1175–1200

Ryan P, Morgan S 2004 Assertive outreach: a strengths approach to policy and practice. Churchill Livingstone, Oxford

Ryan P, Ford R, Beadsmore A et al 1999 The enduring relevance of case management. British Journal of Social Work 29:97–125

Sainsbury Centre for Mental Health 1998 Keys to engagement: review of people with severe mental illness who are hard to engage with services. Sainsbury Centre for Mental Health, London

Satir V 1972 People making. Souvenir Press, London

Sayce L 2000 From psychiatric patient to citizen: overcoming discrimination and social exclusion. Macmillan, London

Schiff A C 2004 Recovery and mental illness: analysis and personal reflections. Psychiatric and Rehabilitation Journal 27(3):212–218

Segal Z V, Williams S, Teasdale J D 2002 Mindfulness-based cognitive therapy for depression: a new approach to preventing relapse. Guilford Press, New York

Seligman M 1975 Helplessness: on depression development and health. Freeman, San Francisco

Seligman M 2002 Authentic happiness. Free Press, New York

Sharpley M, Hutchinson G, McKenzie K, Murray R M 2001 Understanding the excess of psychosis among the African Caribbean population in England. British Journal of Psychiatry Supplement 40:60–68

Silver A, Koehler B, Karon B 2004 Psychodynamic psychotherapy of schizophrenia. In: Read J, Mosher L, Bentall R (eds) Models of madness. Brunner-Routledge, Hove, East Sussex

Smail D 1999 The origins of unhappiness – a new understanding of personal distress. Constable, London

Storr A 1972 The dynamics of creation. Penguin Books, London

Storr A 1988 Solitude. Flamingo/Harper Collins, London

Sullivan H S 1953 The interpersonal theory of psychiatry. W W Norton, New York

Tait L, Birchwood M, Trower P 2003 Predicting engagement with services for psychosis: insight, symptoms and recovery style. British Journal of Psychiatry 182:123–128

Tarrier N, Calam R 2002 New developments in cognitive behavioural case formulation. Epidemiological, systemic and social context: an integrative approach. Behavioural and Cognitive Psychotherapy 30(3):311–328

Tattan T, Tarrier N 2000 The expressed emotion of case managers of the seriously mentally ill. Psychological Medicine 30:195–204

Teall W 2003 The Start model: a profile of using art as a tool in recovery. Available online. http://www.startmc.org.uk (accessed 28 August 2006)

Teall W, Tortora A 2004 Getting to know Alfred Wallis. A Life in the Day 8(3):4–9

Teall W, Tortora A, Cunningham J 2005 Getting to know Alfred Wallis, part 2. Available online. artsednews.squarespace.com/storage/Getting_to_know_Wallis_pt_2.pdf (accessed 28 August 2006)

Thich Nhat Hanh 1991 The miracle of mindfulness. Rider, London

Thich Nhat Hanh 1993 The blooming of a lotus. Beacon Press, Boston

Thomas P, Bracken P 2004 Critical psychiatry in practice. Advances in Psychiatric Treatment 10:361–370

Thorne B 1992 Carl Rogers. Sage Publications, London

Thorne B 1998 Person-centred counselling and Christian spirituality. Whurr, London

Tillich P 2000 The courage to be, 2nd edn. Yale University Press, New Haven

Van Deurzen-Smith E 1988 Existential counselling in practice. Sage Publications, London

Wallcroft J 2000 Becoming fully ourselves. In: Read J, Reynolds J Speaking our minds. Palgrave, Basingstoke

Warner L, Ford R 1998 Conditions for women in in-patient psychiatric units: the Mental Health Act Commission 1996 national visit. Mental Health Care 1(7):225–228

Watkins P 2001 Mental health nursing: the art of compassionate care. Butterworth Heinemann, London

White M 1995 Re-authoring lives: interviews and essays. Dulwich Centre Publications, Adelaide

White M, Epston D 1990 Narrative means to therapeutic ends. W W Norton, New York

Wing J 1970 Institutionalism and schizophrenia. Cambridge University Press, Cambridge

Worden J W 1991 Grief counselling and grief therapy. Springer, New York

Yalom I D 1980 Existential psychotherapy. Basic Books, New York

Zubin J, Spring B 1977 Vulnerability: a new view of schizophrenia. Journal of Abnormal Psychology 86:103–126

Index

Note: Page numbers in italics refer to boxes, figures and tables.

163

165

169